THE NEW PARENTS' GUIDE TO BABY SLEEP TRAINING

LEARN THE SIMPLE SEVEN-DAY SYSTEM FOR ENDING THE SLEEPLESS NIGHTS

By

NATALIE BAKER

CONTENTS

Introduction   v

1. Sleep Training: What It Is and When to   1
   Start
2. Day 1: Establish a Routine   27
3. Day 2: Staying Consistent   53
4. Day 3: Prepare for Tears   79
5. Days 4 and 5: Encourage Healthy Sleep   105
   Patterns
6. Days 6 and 7: The Home Stretch   140

Conclusion   163
References   167

INTRODUCTION

"People who say they sleep like a baby usually don't have one." This famous quote from Leo J. Burke continues to resonate with a lot of parents who are struggling with sleepless nights because of their fussy little ones.

The thing is, sleep problems among babies come in different forms and are due to various reasons. And yet, if you hear a parent share how tough it is to put their baby to sleep, you'd likely find yourself commiserating with them right away.

- Ten-week-old Gabby can fall asleep quickly if she's being rocked to sleep in her mother's arms. Unfortunately, the moment her mom lays her down in the crib, Gabby fusses and cries until someone picks her up again.

- Alice, 8 months old, refuses to go to sleep even when she goes through her usual bedtime routine. She used to be quite cooperative, so it baffles her parents when she suddenly becomes clingier as her bedtime nears.
- At 15 months old, Maria still wakes up two or three times a night. Going back to sleep is impossible for her unless either her mom or dad goes back to her room and sings lullabies to her for up to 30 minutes.

Did any of this sound familiar to you?

Having raised three kids who had their share of sleep issues through the years, I truly understand how exhausting and heartbreaking baby sleep problems can be. It also doesn't help that many parents—especially new ones—tend to second-guess themselves when it comes to dealing with their babies' issues.

It's not just new parents who feel helpless in the face of a crying and screaming baby. Even experienced ones may be shocked when their new babies behave differently than expected. After all, every baby has a unique set of needs and preferences.

So, if you feel like you're doing something wrong to the point of messing up your baby's sleep-wake cycle, know there's a chance that other factors are causing it. It can be hard to remain objective about this when you are on the brink of—or already suffering from—sleep deprivation, but the difficulties of getting your baby to sleep and stay asleep throughout the night can be successfully resolved if you understand what is truly causing the issues.

I remember having these doubts when my children were going through these sleep problems. Taking a deeper look into their sleep habits and schedule led me to more questions about why they could go to sleep as scheduled, or why they woke up cranky or fussy sometimes.

As I delved further, I came across several probable "culprits," such as sleep regression, overtiredness, and separation anxiety. Since your baby might also be going through these issues, I'll share with you what I have learned about them from scientific studies and my personal experiences over the years of raising my children.

Though there are no overnight solutions to the problems and pains brought about by your baby's sleep problems, parents may consider various sleep strategies that have proven to be effective by experts or other parents. Of these strategies, I highly recommend sleep training because it has helped me and my family sleep better throughout the night.

Sleep training has caused quite a stir among parents and experts ever since it was first introduced. While certain methods can be polarizing because they essentially advocate letting babies cry themselves to sleep, some approaches are gentler but still effective. We'll go over the various sleep training methods so that you can better decide which one is suitable for you and your baby.

Case in point, I have sleep-trained my children using different approaches but with great results. Yes, it took me some trial and error to figure things out. But from what I learned in those days, I've come up with a 7-day gradual extinction sleep training plan that may prove to be just as effective at getting you those restful nights your family needs.

Across different chapters of this book, you will learn how to implement this training plan, and I'll supplement those with several actionable tips that can help your baby sleep consistently every night. Other topics that we will cover in this book include:

- Understanding and identifying the reasons for your baby's fussiness and crying
- Selecting the optimal time to begin sleep training your baby and avoiding sensitive age ranges
- Establishing a healthy and sustainable bedtime routine for your baby
- Recognizing the impact of negative sleep associations on your baby's sleep and learning what you can do about them
- Avoiding the common mistakes that parents commit during their baby's sleep training
- Creating a positive bedtime experience for your baby that will encourage the development of healthy sleep patterns

I know this can be quite a lot to take in now—don't worry though because we will discuss everything you need to know one training day at a time. Let my years of experience in sleep training babies serve as your guide and reassurance that your family's sleepless nights will soon come to an end.

You might still have some apprehensions about sleep training at this point. There's no guarantee that it will work for your family too. Here's something to keep in mind as you read through each chapter of this book: Feel free to modify the techniques, schedules, and activity outlines that I will share later. After all, it's best to remain sensitive and responsive to the needs and wants of your family. You're doing this for everyone's sake, so those details must be considered when making and implementing the sleep training plan for your baby.

I'm in my mid-50s now, so my days filled with screaming and crying babies have long passed. Still, I remain passionate about the concept of sleep training because I've seen it work wonders for not just my family, but others who have chosen to use it as well.

It's never too soon—or too late—to start pursuing the goal to improve the way your baby sleeps. With the right set of strategies, lots of patience, and a bit of creativity, you and your family can get all the rest that you deserve.

SLEEP TRAINING: WHAT IT IS AND WHEN TO START

S leep training has always been a controversial topic among parents and child development experts alike. It has been associated with the supposed natural ability of babies to self-soothe, as well as the concept of letting babies cry it out until they fall asleep on their own.

However, much like breastfeeding, vaccination, and other polarizing baby-related issues, sleep training is much more than those assumptions.

In this chapter, I will introduce the concept of sleep training, what it can do for you and your baby, and the ideal timing for it to be effective. We shall also cover the various sleep training methods that are popular among parents to help you better decide which one would best fit your family's needs and preferences.

What Is Sleep Training?

A longitudinal study reported that 50% of the responses from parents stated that their 6-month-old infants woke occasionally in the middle of their sleep, while only 16% indicated that their babies could remain sleeping through the night (Sadler, 1994). Nine percent reported that their babies experience sleep troubles on most nights, and 5% stated that their babies wake up once each night. What's more troubling is that 17% of the respondents said that their babies' sleep tends to get interrupted two to eight times in just one night.

One solution to these sleep interruptions that many child development experts and parents recommend is sleep training. Because of its relative popularity, several variations exist today. The core of these methods, however, is consistent.

Sleep training is all about guiding your baby into learning a healthy sleeping routine that they can carry out with minimal intervention from you or their other caretakers. There is no universal strategy that works for everyone. Instead, it is comprised of various strategies that each have their pros and cons.

Aside from teaching your baby how to fall asleep independently, sleep training also involves applying techniques that can enable your baby to self-soothe and go back to sleep if they suddenly wake up in the middle of the night. Through this, you and other members of your family will not have to wake up as well to put the baby back to sleep.

Given these objectives, the benefits of sleep training will not only be good for your baby, but for everyone responsible for taking care of them at home. After all, multiple research studies have demonstrated the importance of getting enough high-quality sleep, no matter how old you are.

For example, according to a 2007 study conducted by Dr. Ronald E. Dahl of the University of Pittsburg Medical Center, babies should have adequate sleep every night to facilitate the development of critical parts of their brain. Along with proper nutrition and unconditional love and support from their caretakers, sleeping can boost a child's chances of reaching their full potential and become healthy and well-adjusted individuals (Dahl, 2007).

Despite the benefits that you can expect from sleep training your baby, some parents and child development experts do not recommend doing it at all. As mentioned earlier, some methods have certain drawbacks that outweigh the advantages, while other criticisms stem from assumptions and misconceptions about sleep training.

Here are some examples, and why you should not readily believe them:

Sleep training is harsh for babies.

Yes, methods that encourage parents to leave their babies alone when they cry out during sleep training sound cruel for many parents. However, over the past few years, sleep experts have developed other gentler approaches that minimize the harsher aspects of sleep training, such as the Ferber method and the no-tears method.

The great thing about these new methods is that they can still work well even though it may take longer to achieve the objectives of sleep training. As reported by Hiscock et al (2007) in their study about how to improve the quality of sleep among babies and the mental health of their mothers, parents who utilized gentler sleep training methods reported 30%

fewer sleep problems with their babies in the five months after they completed the training.

Sleep training causes long-term damage to children.

No objective data exists to support this claim at the moment. Conversely, there is also no research data indicating that skipping sleep training will result in developmental problems later on.

Therefore, you should not feel pressured to either go through or avoid sleep training your child. Your decision about this matter should depend largely on the current needs and preferences of your baby, and the general well-being of you and your family.

Progress can only be measured by the amount of crying your baby will do during sleep training.

Not at all! What you should be monitoring is the overall response of your baby toward the sleep training method you have chosen. Did your baby become fussier? Is your baby affected whenever you check in on them? Should you stick to reassuring words instead of gentle pats to soothe your baby?

While less crying indicates that extinction-based methods are working, you don't have to rely solely on that to know if sleep training is effective for your baby. For example, in the no-tears approach, you can measure the length of time it takes for your baby to feel drowsy and fall asleep as you fade out their current sleeping habits.

Once you have sleep-trained your baby, you won't have to ever worry about the quality and length of their sleep again.

None of the sleep training methods available today can accomplish that feat. Many parents stand by certain methods because they got the results that they wanted. However, do not discount the instances where the result lasted for only a short term.

In such cases, parents may opt to try out other sleep training methods and see if those will work better. It is best to consult the child's pediatrician to better understand other choices that you can explore.

Various factors also affect the quality and duration of a baby's sleep. Sometimes, no matter how well you have trained your baby, they can still have a restless night because they are suffering from an illness, or were too stimulated during the day. In times like these, there is nothing you can do but be there for your infant and try your best to help them fall and stay asleep.

Again, sleep training is not considered an essential parenting strategy for everyone. You are free to decide whether to apply its techniques to develop and improve your baby's sleeping habits. Many parents who opted out of sleep training reported that their children learned how to fall asleep and stay asleep without intervention or training.

However, if you decide to try to sleep train your baby, remember to consult a pediatrician first, as well as other members of your family. Professional opinions are a necessity since sleep training could affect your child's health and development. Keep in mind that the ideal sleep training approach for your baby is both doable and accepted by the other family members participating.

As you will learn later in this book, sleep training is not something that you can or should do on your own. Having the support and cooperation of the other people who take care of your baby will increase the effectiveness and ensure the steady progress of sleep training.

When Should You Start Sleep Training Your Baby?

Several sleep training experts say that the best time to sleep train a baby is when they are between 4 and 6 months old.

At this point, the baby has the right set of cognitive skills and personal abilities that enables them to soothe themselves and absorb the sleep techniques that you are trying to teach. Moreover, the babies' feeding times tend to be spaced out more, thus allowing them to sleep for six to eight hours without feeling the need to wake up due to hunger.

This is further explained in the book entitled "Bedtiming: The Parent's Guide to Getting Your Child to Sleep at Just the Right Age" (Lewis & Granic, 2010). It outlines the conditions that might affect the effectiveness of the training according to age range, but bear in mind that these are not fixed and may vary from one baby to another.

Newborn to 2.5 Months

Babies who fall under this category cannot differentiate yet between day and night. Aside from the lack of conscious awareness about their surroundings, they also do not produce melatonin—a hormone produced in the brain as a response to the presence or absence of light.

Newborns also require frequent feeding, regardless of whether it is breastmilk or formula. This continues up until somewhere between their second or third month of age. In most cases, babies wake up on their own whenever they feel hunger. However, some babies need to be woken up in the middle of their sleep just so they can follow a healthy feeding schedule.

Because of this, attempting to introduce sleeping techniques to newborns, and particularly young babies, is not recommended. Let your baby follow their instincts when it comes to sleeping and feeding and try your best to accommodate and fulfill those needs.

3 to 4 Months

By this age, babies are starting to adapt to a natural circadian rhythm. You should notice that their wake-up times and sleeping times cycle at a more even pace. This is going to form a critical part of the foundation of your child's sleep training.

In their third and fourth month of age, most babies tend to feel more comfortable and secure even when they are left on their own. However, do not expect them to be able to soothe themselves if they become irritated or hungry to the point of waking up during their sleep. Because of this, many parents still find this age range to be a difficult point to start sleep training their babies.

4.5 to 5.5 Months

Much of the sweet spot for sleep training is within this age range. Babies have become more accustomed to regular sleep-wake cycles, so teaching them about various sleeping techniques should be a lot easier.

At this age, your baby will also likely sleep for around six to eight hours straight each night. Their feeding schedule does not require them to wake up or be woken up at some point during their sleep, thus minimizing the probable effects of sleep training on their health and development.

However, many parents experience challenges when it comes to crying episodes. They notice that babies who fall under this age range are learning how effective crying can be at gaining their parents' attention.

Tears are purely emotional or instinctual reactions, but are also something that they can use to get their desired response from the people around them. Therefore, parents who plan to begin sleep training their babies at this age should also equip themselves with strategies on how to manage these crying episodes.

6 to 8 Months

Many parents and sleep training experts find this period to be suitable, too. Babies are still receptive to being taught about sleeping techniques and self-soothing methods. It helps that they also tend to be less fussy at this point, even when their sleep gets interrupted before their regular waking time.

Do note that most babies who belong to this age range typically pay more attention to their toys and other favorite objects than their caretakers. Take this into account when you are deciding on which sleep training method you will choose for your baby.

9 to 11 Months

By your baby's ninth to the eleventh month of age, they will likely experience less separation anxiety, especially during bedtime. As Dr. Granic explained in her book, babies in this age range start to learn that their parents are not permanently leaving them when they are left behind in the room.

However, this may pose a challenge as well, since your baby will also start to notice that you are going to pay attention to them even when they cannot see you. As such, expect to have more crying episodes if you choose to start sleep training for your baby within this period of their development.

12 to 16 Months

As your baby becomes a toddler, their focus will shift more to gaining and improving their communication skills and various abilities. Therefore, your child may exhibit less clingy tendencies toward you and their other caretakers.

Since they are eager to learn and are starting to be more independent, this could also be a great time to begin their sleep training. As you will learn in the succeeding section of this chapter, some sleep training methods work better when your child is within this age range or older.

17 to 21 Months

If you have not yet attempted to sleep train your child before this age, continue putting off the training, and allow your child enough time and space to learn and adapt a good sleeping routine on their own.

Otherwise, you might hamper the development of their growing self-confidence and independence. Experts noted that toddlers in this age range may regress to their needy selves if their parents pay too much attention to everything they do.

Intervene only if you notice that your child continues to experience troubles in falling asleep and staying asleep throughout the night. At that point, seek the professional opinion of a pediatrician before deciding on a sleep training strategy for your child.

Though you should pay attention to what sleep training experts and other parents say about the ideal timing for babies, feel free to consider doing it regardless of your baby's age. Infants develop at different rates. Others might be ready for training at an earlier age, while some would be more receptive to it if their parents waited a little longer.

In some cases, parents cannot apply sleep training techniques even if they wanted to. For example, Carla and Dan had to delay sleep training their daughter Emily until they had moved to their new house.

Why?

The sleep training method they believed would work well with Emily required her to have a separate bedroom from her parents. As such, their family started sleep training when Emily was already 12 months old.

You might assume that at that point, the baby has already developed sleeping habits that could be hard to shake off, but as attested to by many parents like Carla and Dan, timing does not matter much if you can still reach your goals for sleep training your baby.

How Can You Sleep Train Your Baby?

Various sleep training methods have been developed by experts over the years. Some are rooted in classic pieces of advice that are passed down from one generation to another, while others stem from more recent studies about the behavior and cognitive abilities of infants and toddlers.

As explained earlier, none of these methods can guarantee total success in terms of establishing a healthy and sustainable sleeping routine for babies. However, each of them has its own set of pros and cons that could be more suitable for your child's needs and preferences, as well as for the achievement of your sleep training objectives.

To help you evaluate and select a sleep training approach for your child, below is a rundown of six methods that are popular and trusted by many parents:

No-Tears Method

As championed by sleep training expert Elizabeth Pantley, this method aims to gradually change a baby's sleeping habits to minimize crying as they learn to sleep on their own. As such, many also refer to this as the No-Cry method.

Two techniques are commonly associated with this method. First is the so-called "fading" trick. To do this, you must lessen the association of a particular habit with your baby's sleep up to the point wherein your baby no longer has to rely on that habit to fall asleep.

For example, if you normally rock your baby in your arms until they fall asleep, you should slowly reduce the duration of your rocking each night. You have succeeded in fading out this habit if your baby could fall asleep without being rocked in your arms at all.

The other technique that could help you achieve the objectives of the no-tears method is substitution. Pantley explains that babies may be weaned gently and more easily away from their sleep habits if you could substitute the said habits with a weaker sleep association.

Sounds confusing?

It's quite simple. For instance, if your baby typically falls asleep after being nursed, consider substituting nursing with rocking instead. Give your baby enough time to get used to being rocked to sleep, and then work on gradually fading out rocking. Since it is a relatively new sleeping habit, you would find it easier to wean your baby away from this sleep association than nursing, which you have likely done for your baby for a far longer time.

Cry It Out (CIO) Method

Also known as full extinction or extinction, this method is based on the scientific theory that behavioral tendencies may be phased out by not responding to them.

In the context of bedtime routines, it means letting your baby fall asleep on their own even if they start to cry. After all, some studies—such as the longitudinal intervention study conducted by Burnham, Goodlin-Jones, Gaylor, and Anders (2002)—have shown that babies may be taught, or may learn on their own, the ability to self-soothe.

By instinct, most parents respond to crying by attempting to pacify their children right away. However, this could reinforce an unwanted behavior since your child is essentially getting a good response or even a reward just because they cried.

Given this, the CIO method suggests the following basic steps for sleep training your baby:

1. Make sure that your baby is well-fed, clean, and comfortable.
2. Tuck your baby into their crib while they are still awake.
3. Leave your baby in their bedroom after saying goodnight.
4. Refrain from going back or responding in any way to your baby, even if they started crying.
5. Return to your baby's room at their supposed wake-up time, or at their pre-determined feeding times.

As a parent myself, being told that the best way to sleep train your baby is by ignoring their cries can be hard to accept. Such sentiment is echoed by many parents, caretakers, and even some sleep training experts. After all, while hearing your baby cry for a long time can be quite a distressful experience, imagine how helpless and emotionally worn out your baby will be throughout the night.

However, the good thing about the CIO method is its speed in terms of your baby's progress in learning how to fall asleep and stay asleep regularly. Yes, the first two nights would likely be rough for both you and your baby. Fortunately, by the third and fourth nights, many parents have reported significant improvements and less crying.

The key to achieving this is consistency. This means exercising self-control by not interfering with the process even when you hear your child crying out because they cannot fall asleep or because they have suddenly been woken up.

Weissbluth Method

As popularized by Dr. Marc Weissbluth in his book "Healthy Sleep Habits, Happy Child" (2015), this method combines the theory behind extinction with the benefits of following a good sleeping routine for your baby. As such, its process bears a lot of similarities with the CIO method, as outlined above.

However, rather than simply putting the baby in the crib and leaving the room after saying goodnight, parents should establish and consistently go through a bedtime routine with their baby. Popular examples of activities that may be part of a good bedtime routine include giving the baby a nice, warm bath, reading a children's book, and singing or listening to a lullaby. Because of the additional step, the Weissbluth method recommends starting the bedtime routine earlier than other sleep training methods do.

Some people confuse the Weissbluth method with the Ferber method. This stems from the part wherein the baby learns to sleep better when they figure out how to self-soothe when they fuss or cry. The difference between the two can be observed in the required pacing and amount of intervention that parents may do during the process.

When done properly, you may see significant results from doing the Weissbluth method as quickly as with the CIO method. However, be prepared for emotional distress because, unless there is an emergency, you are not allowed to return to your baby's room or try in any way to soothe your baby when they become fussy or cry out. In comparison, the Ferber method has a more gradual pace, but it allows parents to comfort their babies at regular intervals throughout the night.

Ferber Method

Developed and popularized by Dr. Richard Ferber, this method is a gentler variation of the extinction technique. As such, some people refer to it as the "timed-interval sleep training," "check-and-console method," or "gradual extinction sleep training."

The goal of the Ferber method is to teach the baby to sleep on their own. However, rather than leaving the baby alone throughout the night, parents are allowed to check in at predetermined time intervals and offer some degree of comfort to the baby as needed.

Take for example how I applied this method to my babies. During the first night, I went through the normal bedtime routine of my baby. While he was still awake, I put him down in the crib and then left the room for a minute.

Once the set time lapsed, I returned to the room and gave reassurance to my baby through gentle pats or words. Picking up and holding my baby in my arms is not allowed by the Ferber method so I refrained from doing so.

The cycle of leaving and returning continued until my baby had fallen asleep. Take note that the time interval for each cycle must be gradually increased to about 10 to 15 minutes. If my baby woke up in the middle of his sleep, I started the Ferber method over to put him back to sleep.

For many parents who have followed this method, they noticed that their objectives for sleep training could be achieved within one week—though there have been cases where it took the parents around two weeks instead.

During the first couple of nights, you might not see significant progress, so experts recommend writing down your observations in a sleep-training log. Through this log, you can objectively evaluate if the Ferber method is working for your child or not.

Chair Method

As its name implies, this method involves sitting down on a chair beside your baby's crib as they fall asleep, and then leaving your baby alone unless you notice that they have woken up again. With each night that passes, the chair must be gradually moved further away from the crib until you are not in your baby's room anymore as they try to go to sleep on their own.

Other terms used for this sleep training technique include "gradual withdrawal" and "sleep lady shuffle." Some parents and sleep training experts stand by this method because it eases the baby into good sleeping habits. Because of that, the process takes a bit longer to complete; most implementation plans last for at least two weeks.

Moreover, parents following this method have the option to soothe or calm their babies when needed, since they are present in the room. Some experts allow touching and patting the baby, but in general, parents should try their best to refrain from intervening, even if the baby is crying out or having trouble with their sleep.

A lot of parents find this hard to consistently implement. After all, seeing your baby in distress would likely spur you on to act immediately. Your baby might cry even more to get your attention.

By not responding to them, you could cause some confusion for your child, especially if they are too young to recognize that extending or escalating their cries would not give them what they want. In some cases, this may also cause overstimulation, thus preventing them from calming themselves down on their own.

Pick-Up-Put-Down Method

This training method allows parents to check on their sleeping infants at regular intervals, and to give comfort if needed. This may sound like the Ferber method, but the difference is in terms of what kind of comfort may be offered to the baby.

Parents who apply this method are allowed to pick up their babies and hold them in their arms for a few minutes. In theory, the baby should be sufficiently calmed down by the time they are put back in the crib. As a result, they should feel drowsy and return to sleep on their own.

Which Sleep Training Method Should You Apply?

Having learned the various ways to sleep train your baby, it is likely that you have at least one in mind that you think would be a good fit for everyone involved. Remember to check with your baby's pediatrician, and to discuss the options with your family and the other caretakers of your baby.

"First thing in the morning, we're really tired, and we look at each other and we wonder, 'Are we ever going to get sleep?' And yet, it doesn't matter if you don't get sleep. It's an honor to take care of them."

— ANGELINA JOLIE

An important factor that must be considered when choosing a sleep training method is the age and rate of development of your infant. Certain sleep training methods work better among younger babies —for example, the pick-up-put-down method. These infants prefer to feel the presence of their parents, while older babies might feel too stimulated by being picked up and held when they should be trying to fall asleep again.

For older babies and toddlers, some experts have noted that the chair method is more effective than when it is applied at a younger age. At the latter part of your baby's development, they are beginning to fully grasp the idea that not seeing you for several minutes or hours does not mean that you have completely abandoned them.

Parents who are after quick results pick either the CIO method or the Weissbluth method. However, these sleep training strategies require a lot more than consistency and mental fortitude to be successfully carried out. You will also need to set up a separate bedroom for your baby. The Weissbluth method may also be too much for some parents to handle since it will essentially prevent them from socializing or leaving the house by early evening.

If you can't stand the thought of your child crying for extended periods like the extinction-based strategies allow, then your go-to strategy would be the no-tears method. Be prepared to spend time gradually fading out or substituting the sleep habits of your baby though. Since progress is expected to be much slower, you need to be patient and consistent throughout the process.

I always recommend new parents try the gradual extinction strategy. While it still involves letting your child cry, it does not force babies to learn self-soothing on their own. Parents may opt to provide comfort and reassurance to their distressed babies, thus reducing the emotional impact that sleep training could cause on everyone involved.

Given these reasons, the rest of this book will focus more on guiding you on how to properly implement the gradual extinction strategy for sleep training your baby. So, prepare your sleep-training log, and next I'll show you step-by-step how to start your baby's sleep training with gradual extinction.

2

DAY 1: ESTABLISH A ROUTINE

As discussed in the previous chapter, one of the most critical components of successfully sleep training a baby is consistency. For extinction-based methods, you need to be consistent in leaving your child alone during their bedtime. Otherwise, your baby would take longer to adjust, thus prolonging their distressful nights.

On the other hand, gentler methods—such as fading and substitution—require parents to be consistent in easing their infants away from their bad sleep associations. Habits can be especially hard to break if you just fall back into doing them again "once in a while."

Parents who follow the gradual extinction strategy must be consistent. This can be achieved by guiding your baby to sleep through a bedtime routine every night.

Therefore, your goal for the first day of sleep training is to establish a healthy bedtime routine that works for everyone. In this chapter, I will demonstrate to you how important it is to get this right, and what you should do to achieve your first goal in sleep training your baby.

The Importance of Establishing a Bedtime Routine

To come up with a good bedtime routine for your baby, you need to be sensitive to their needs and preferences. It takes time, energy, and patience to create one, and even more once you have to actually carry out the routine.

But why go through this much effort? What can your baby gain from having an established bedtime routine? Can you also benefit from it somehow?

According to an article posted by Pacheco (2021), the benefits of a bedtime routine are as follows:

- Bedtime routines can calm down and relax the baby's body and mind. If your baby has had an exciting or emotion-filled day, going through their regular bedtime routine could help ease away the adrenaline or agitation from their system.
- Babies who follow a bedtime routine tend to fall asleep quicker and stay asleep longer than those who don't. Moreover, they are less affected by factors that may cause their sleep to be interrupted, such as sudden noises or movements near their sleeping area.
- Higher quality of sleep leads to the improvement of certain cognitive skills, such as working memory and attention. As such, babies who got sufficient high-quality sleep with the help of an established bedtime routine will likely grow up to reach their maximum potential, especially in terms of skills development and academic performance.
- Bedtime routines can strengthen the bond between the baby and their parents. It is an opportunity to spend quality time together.

Parents should take this chance to be caring and give undivided attention to their babies.

- A baby's bedtime routine can be a time for parents to relax too. When selecting activities that will be included in the routine, consider what you will also find enjoyable and calming. This makes it easier for you to keep doing the bedtime routine until your baby has fully accepted it.

As you can see, the positive effects of bedtime routines for your baby can be felt in different aspects of their development. It also serves as one of the pillars of your child's healthy habits that they can bring with them as they grow up and become more independent.

When Should You Do It?

Babies can learn and adapt to a new and healthier bedtime routine by the time they are six to eight weeks old. Beginning earlier than this would likely put pressure on you and your baby when both of you should be recovering from their birth.

The natural circadian rhythm is not yet in place among younger babies. As such, their nighttime patterns are largely dictated by other bodily factors, such as hunger and irritation from soiled diapers.

On the other hand, most babies who are within six to eight weeks of age have a better sense of day and night. They naturally feel drowsy when nighttime approaches, and with your guidance, they can be taught to fall asleep on schedule through a bedtime routine.

Another signal that your baby needs a bedtime routine is when they begin to become dependent on "sleep aids," These pertain to the unsustainable actions that parents usually do just to make their babies fall asleep. Common examples of sleep aids include:

- Nursing the baby to sleep
- Cradling the baby in your arms while they sleep
- Letting the baby fall asleep while sucking on a pacifier

"There are hard days in motherhood. But looking at your sleeping baby reminds you why it's all worth it."

— KARA FERWERDA

Sleep aids can be quite helpful for younger babies who cannot be taught a bedtime routine yet. However, once your baby is of the appropriate age, wean them off of these sleep aids because you can't always carry or rock your baby in your arms until they are asleep. Baby pacifiers can also harm your child in the long run. Rather than relying on these sleep aids, replace them with a bedtime routine that can help them fall asleep on their own as they grow older.

Establishing a bedtime routine is also necessary if there will be big changes in your schedule as well. Parents who plan to go back to work, for instance, should work on this so they will also have enough time to rest and sleep themselves. A baby who can sleep and stay asleep throughout the night makes it a lot easier for the rest of the family to get back to their day-to-day routines and handle their responsibilities in other aspects of their lives.

Before You Start

Anything important requires a plan. Sleep training your little one certainly counts as an important project. Without thinking things over before you start, you might subject yourself, your child, and other members of your family, to several distressful nights that would amount to nothing in the end. That is why you should pay careful attention to the five tips given below to ensure that you start out on the right foot with your journey toward restful sleep for everyone in the family.

1. Try to get as much rest and sleep as you can. Regardless of which sleep training method you choose, expect things to be exhausting—physically, mentally, and emotionally—once you begin.

2. Prepare a log of your baby's sleeping schedule and patterns.A sleep log based on the current bedtime habits and sleep duration of your baby will help you to make key decisions.

First, it can tell you the ideal schedule for sleep training your baby. The sleep log indicates the start and end of the various activities that your baby does

throughout the day and night, such as playing, feeding, napping, and sleeping. You can do this in a
spreadsheet file, or if you prefer a manual approach,
keep a notebook listing their activities and the time
they happen during the day.

Another benefit of having a sleep log is that it can
serve as a reference for you and your infant's pediatrician. For example, some babies have trouble
sleeping because of their inconsistent or incompat-
ible feeding schedules. Going through the contents
of the sleep log may help parents and pediatricians
to recognize or rule out this possibility.

Maintain a sleep log for at least two weeks before
your planned starting day for sleep training. This
should give you enough time to gather sufficient
information that will be valuable in choosing and
implementing the right sleep training method for
your baby.

3. Consult your baby's pediatrician.

Quick Tip!

Color code your baby's sleep log to make it easier for
you to spot and understand their sleeping patterns
and schedule. Assign different colors for each

activity and use that as a reference when recording your baby's activities in the sleep log.

Your primary reason for doing this is to eliminate any possibility that your infant's sleeping trouble is caused by an underlying medical issue. For example, it may be due to something as natural as teething, or something as serious as sleep apnea.

Parents are highly discouraged from relying on their observations alone, since babies require specialized care and attention from medical professionals. You can look for the common signs associated with conditions that could be interfering with your baby's sleep, log them, and discuss them with your doctor.

Remember to bring your baby's sleep log when you go for a consultation. Discuss the patterns and habits that you have recognized, and keep an open mind about your pediatrician's observations, too. A fresh set of eyes may be able to point out something important that you have missed.

"Lack of direction, not lack of time, is the problem. We all have twenty-four hour days."

— ZIG ZIGLAR

4. Form your plan.

Now that you have a good idea about what should be done to address your infant's sleep troubles, use that knowledge to decide how you will sleep train your baby. This should be centered on the method you have chosen, as well as the optimal schedule for everyone involved.

Create an outline of the steps that you will undertake, including the activities that will form part of your baby's bedtime routine. Consider going the extra mile by setting some guidelines on how the sleep training strategy should be carried out by you, and the responsibilities of other members of the family. Remember to establish the do's and don'ts so that everyone will be on the same page.

Write down your plan and put it up somewhere that is accessible for everyone helping you sleep train your baby. This will serve as a reference and reminder, so try to strike a balance between being informative and being concise.

Sleep training experts recommend having at least a one-week plan. This will be enough to determine whether the selected strategy is effective for your baby. Do note that your plan may still be adjusted as needed. If you believe that your plan is causing significant distress or harm to your baby or anyone else in the family, you are free to stop the training and make a new plan that works for everyone.

5. Clear your schedule.

As explained in the previous chapter, sleep training will likely take up a significant portion of your time and energy, especially because during the same time you should be getting rest and sleep yourself. To make things easier for everyone involved, try your best to clear your calendar for at least the next two weeks before beginning your baby's sleep training.

This can prevent you from putting too much on your plate at one time, ensuring that you can keep focused on what must be done to guide your baby into falling and staying asleep on their own.

Most importantly, clearing your schedule will help you remain consistent throughout the process. After all, following the bedtime routine that you have established for your baby can be quite difficult if your days or nights are filled with other obligations and commitments.

Recommended Activities for the Bedtime Routine for Your Baby

Though no universal bedtime routine can work for every infant, some routines have been tried and tested by many parents in terms of how effective they are in relaxing and lulling their babies to sleep. The key, however, is not simply replicating these routines, but figuring out which bedtime routine activity would be suitable and doable for both you and your baby.

Therefore, to help you come up with a bedtime routine, check out this list of recommended activities that could form a part of your little one's bedtime routine.

Feeding

Depending on your baby's age, doing this can lessen the chance of their sleep being interrupted in the middle of the night just because they are feeling hungry. Since younger babies require more frequent feeding, this particular benefit applies more to those who are at least 12 months old or older.

You don't have to limit your baby to just breastmilk or formula. If they can already eat solid foods, something light but nutritious would be a great nighttime snack for your baby—for example, porridge and rice pudding.

Remember to wipe your baby's gums or brush their teeth once feeding time is over. If you notice that they tend to fall asleep while feeding, schedule it earlier so they don't become dependent on this as a sleep aid.

Giving a gentle massage

Studies show that babies sleep better after being gently massaged before bedtime (Nahidi et al, 2017).

Why?

It's mostly because the rubbing motion stimulates the production of melatonin—a body hormone that is necessary to fall asleep faster and to remain asleep throughout the night. Massaging your baby can also soothe some pains and discomfort that could prevent them from falling asleep, such as stomach aches and teething pains.

Infant massage can be a great opportunity to strengthen the bond between you and your baby. Of all the senses, touch is usually the one that develops the earliest, so most babies can already appreciate the gentle strokes and rubs from others.

Furthermore, giving a massage to babies can be quite relaxing for their parents, too. Just remember to pay close attention to your baby's cues to tell if they are enjoying it or not. If you notice that your baby is shying away, frowning, or crying when you attempt to give them a massage, stop what you are doing for now, and try again at some other time and with other massage techniques.

Giving a relaxing bath

For this to be effective, remember to use warm water and mild soap for your baby. Look for something that is either lavender- or chamomile-scented since those have been proven to be quite relaxing, even among infants.

Take note that several pediatricians do not suggest a nightly bath for babies, especially newborns, because it may cause their delicate skin to dry out and become irritated.

Changing their clothes

No one can sleep well if their clothes are dirty and sticky. As such, your baby will fall asleep faster and stay asleep longer if you change their clothes to appropriate sleepwear every night. It's not as simple as it sounds though.

Many parents believe that babies should sleep with one additional layer than what they wear during the day. However, this rule of thumb does not necessarily apply to every situation.

An overly dressed infant may suffer from overheating, which could then increase the risk of Sudden Infant Death Syndrome (SIDS)—which refers to the unexpected and unexplainable deaths of babies, typically during their sleep. Therefore, remember to stick to light but snug sleeping clothes, especially during summer.

Reading a book

Most babies, even newborns, enjoy this activity. Though they cannot understand the words or the plot yet, listening to the voices of their parents can be an incredibly soothing way to bond.

Select books that have good rhyme and repetition. Be gentle and speak slowly so that your baby can better appreciate the sounds that you are making.

Brightly colored books that have special touch-and-feel features can also be great for bedtime. Encourage your little one to reach out and touch as you read to them. If your baby is 12 months old or older, consider telling stories about your experiences, favorite moments, or even about some fun character you just made up.

Listening to a lullaby or white noise

Some parents believe that it is best to sing rather than simply play or stream a lullaby for their baby. While it can be a good bonding moment, singing may be considered to be a sleep aid since there is no guarantee that you will always have the energy or be in the mood for this.

That is why many sleep experts suggest playing or streaming lullabies instead if it is going to be a part of a baby's sleep routine. Select gentle songs that have around 60 beats per minute because faster songs can just excite the baby, having the opposite effect of what you are going for.

Aside from lullabies, listening to white noise can be comforting and relaxing for babies because it resembles the sounds that they were hearing while they were still in the womb. White noise machines can easily be purchased nowadays, even ones that are specifically designed to promote sleep among infants.

Saying goodnight

Think of reassuring parting words that you could say every night before leaving your baby's room. Keep it short and sweet—something like "Good night, little one" or "Mommy/Daddy loves you."

Make these words extra effective by coupling them with caring gestures, like a soft pat on their cheek or a gentle kiss on their forehead.

Take time to reflect on each activity and feel free to try out some of them to see how your baby responds.

Helpful Tips on Establishing Your Baby's Bedtime Routine

Since this is likely your first time preparing a bedtime routine for your baby, I'm sharing with you eight tips that you should seriously consider to ensure that the first day of sleep training your baby will be a success:

Tip #1: Keep it simple.

The bedtime routine should be something that you can easily do every night. It should not be too complicated to the point that you don't feel relaxed. Otherwise, your baby will likely notice your distress or worry thus further preventing them from falling asleep themselves.

Create a routine that you can also perform even if you and your baby are not at home. Whether your family is staying for the night at someone else's house or in a hotel during a trip, the bedtime routine of your baby must remain consistent as much as possible.

Tip #2: Time it right.

Remember the sleep log you prepared before Day 1 of sleep training? Use that in setting the initial schedule for your baby's bedtime routine. Look for the times where your baby has slept the longest and with the least sleep interruption.

Time the start of the bedtime routine at least 30 minutes from the target bedtime of your little one.

For example, if you aim to get your baby to sleep by 8 p.m., initiate the bedtime routine by 7:30 p.m.

On average, this would be enough time for you to complete the entire routine without rushing your way through it. Feel free to adjust the duration though, depending on the actual bedtime routine of your baby.

Tip #3: Location is key.

A lot of babies, especially younger ones, fall asleep while they are in their strollers, car seats, or swings. That is fine, but try your best to transfer them as soon as possible to their crib.

If an errand would coincide with your baby's naptime, avoid bringing them along with you as much as possible. Refrain from scheduling errands during that period. For times that it can't be helped (we all live in the real world), move your sleeping baby to their crib once you have returned home.

Tip #4: Create the ideal atmosphere for sleeping.

Exposing your baby to bright lights or screens during bedtime will throw off their natural circadian rhythm. Therefore, you should dim the lights in their bedroom. If possible, turn off the overhead lights and stick to night lights instead.

If bright lights from the outside stream through the window, draw the curtains or blinds closed. That will also help muffle some of the outside sounds that may disrupt your baby's sleep.

Turn off the television or computer before bedtime. Remember to put your cellphone or other personal mobile devices in either silent or vibrate mode.

Be mindful of the temperature of your baby's bedroom. If it's too cold, your baby will likely wake up more frequently. On the other hand, high temperature increases the risk of SIDS. Experts suggest maintaining the room temperature between 68°F (20°C) and 72°F (22°C) throughout the night.

Tip #5: Pay attention to the sleep cues of your baby.

Sleep cues refer to the behaviors that indicate tiredness or drowsiness, such as yawning, rubbing their face, or looking away. The best time to observe and learn your baby's sleeping cues is during their first four months after birth. At this point, they do not follow a regular sleeping schedule yet, so pay attention to what your baby usually does before they sleep.

Some sleep cues can easily be spotted, but some may be too subtle for parents to notice without prior knowledge of what to look for. This will be discussed in the next chapter since learning how to recognize and handle these sleep cues is critical for staying consistent with the bedtime routine.

If you notice that your baby is exhibiting their sleep cues, soothe them right away because ignoring these cues may lead to fussiness or crying. If their tiredness escalates to that point, it will take your baby much longer to fall asleep.

Tip #6: Reassure your baby.

Bedtimes can be quite stressful for many babies because it separates them from their parents. Younger babies do not yet understand what happens once you leave the room. As a result, they may fuss or cry to get your attention back on them.

A bedtime routine that lasts for about 10 to 30 minutes will likely be enough to relieve your baby of their separation anxiety. During this time, try your best to reassure your baby that you love and care for them. Show it through gentle actions that will calm their thoughts and emotions. Make sure to do this in their sleeping area though so that they will associate these reassuring gestures with that space and the idea that they will be left alone afterward.

Tip #7: Anticipate some resistance from your child.

When it comes to bedtime routines, more resistance can be expected from older babies and toddlers. This comes in different forms, such as requesting more reading time or finding some fault in the pajamas they are wearing.

The reasons vary from one child to another, but their goal is common: to delay bedtime as much as possible. Handling your little one's resistance will be easier once you know the type of resistance to expect.

Be observant about the points in the bedtime routine where your child tends to act up. You might be tempted to give in to their request, especially if you think it is reasonable, but that may prevent them from fully embracing their bedtime routine. Rather than simply acquiesce, be firm yet gentle in turning down their attempts to delay and try your best to explain to your little one why they should follow the routine.

Tip #8: Create a naptime routine for your baby.

Aside from helping you stay on schedule when it comes to your baby's naptimes, doing this will also further strengthen the sleep cues that you have introduced in the bedtime routine. As a result, your baby will accept these cues quicker, which will then allow them to fall asleep faster and more consistently.

Base the naptime routine on the bedtime routine you have established. You may shorten it though since naps are also shorter but more frequent than sleeping at night. Select the sleep cues that seem to be quite effective for your baby and incorporate them together into a 10- to 15-minute naptime routine.

As you can see, establishing your baby's bedtime routine involves careful thought and planning for it to be effective. The great thing is that all of these are doable and applicable for most cases. However, if you believe that something else would work better for you, your baby, or the other members of your family, feel free to use your ideas as long as you can continue to monitor things closely.

Adjustment to bedtime may also be needed as your baby grows older. Something that they like doing now might not be as enjoyable as time goes on.

You might also have to adjust the time of certain activities when your baby becomes older. For example, my son used to find baths incredibly relaxing when he was 6 months old. As such, I included it in his regular bedtime routine. However, by the time he reached his twelfth month, bath time before bed had become a playful affair so I had to move it further away from his supposed bedtime.

Suggested Bedtime Routine for Day 1

To better demonstrate what a bedtime routine should look like, I'm sharing the bedtime routine that I established for my first-born son on Day 1 of his sleep training.

Back then, I allotted one hour for the entire bedtime routine. The exact time varied depending on the kind of day he had—for instance, it would be shorter if he had exhausted himself during playtime.

The time can also be different depending on the temperament of your baby. Some are quite excitable and tend to require longer bedtime routines, while babies who are more low-key are usually faster to be lulled into sleep.

Given these factors, take the following outline as a guide, not a fixed schedule that is guaranteed to be just as effective for your baby. Use this as a reference for the kind of activities that you should consider for the bedtime routine of your little one, and feel free to tweak it according to what you believe would work for your family.

- 1 hour before bedtime
- Give your baby a bath using warm water and a mild lavender-scented body wash.
- Change their diaper to a clean one.
- Gently apply baby lotion all over their body, arms, and legs.
- 45 minutes before bedtime
- Perform a quick infant massage.
- Dress your baby in clean sleeping clothes.
- Turn on a piece of soothing background music or white noise.
- Dim the lights in your baby's bedroom.
- 30 minutes before bedtime

- Feed or nurse your baby.
- Read, listen to a lullaby, or perform any calming activity that you and your little one enjoy.
- 10 minutes before bedtime
- Burp your baby, if needed.
- Snuggle or gently rock them in your arms.
- 5 minutes before bedtime
- Put your baby into the crib while they are still awake.
- Tuck them in with a blanket, if needed.
- Reassure them with words, a soft kiss, and/or gentle touches.
- Bedtime
- Leave the bedroom quietly.
- Do not return until the next timed interval or until their supposed wake-up time.

Once you have successfully established your baby's bedtime routine, your next goal in sleep training, via the gradual extinction strategy, is to follow through and remain consistent. Doing so will ensure that the hard work you have done so far does not go to waste. In the next chapter we discuss how you can accomplish this during the second day of your baby's sleep training.

3

DAY 2: STAYING CONSISTENT

A good bedtime routine for your baby will mean nothing if you can't stick to it. Without consistency, you are just going to waste the time and energy of everyone involved in sleep training your baby. Both you and your little one will end up suffering more sleepless nights since you will be thrown back to step one every time you fail to follow through with the bedtime routine. For those reasons, your goal for Day 2 of sleep training is to stay consistent.

Various factors may make this goal harder to achieve. Of these, schedule, exhaustion, and hearing your baby cry out tend to be the biggest hurdles for many parents.

Getting the timing right for your baby's bedtime can be tricky, especially if it is your first attempt to sleep train them. You must try! A healthy bedtime routine involves putting your baby to sleep when they are tired and drowsy enough to go to sleep. Any sooner than that, your baby will likely miss their supposed sleeping time. On the other hand, delays in the bedtime routine can lead to overtiredness—a state which may sound like something that would help your baby sleep faster and better. But, as you will learn later in this book, overtiredness will prevent your baby from being sleep trained successfully.

To help you figure out the optimal scheduled bedtime for your baby, this chapter will go over the common signs of tiredness that can be observed among babies from different age groups.

Putting your baby to bed at the right time will allow you to stay on track with your baby's bedtime routine. This can become quite exhausting for both you and your baby, especially since it will likely entail many adjustments to your routine. It's not just your baby who might feel overtired during sleep training—you may find yourself feeling so tired that you cannot push yourself to go through your baby's bedtime routine.

Inconsistency due to exhaustion will become a bigger hurdle for parents if they hear their baby crying. Depending on their age, changes in their usual nighttime activities

---

"Consistent actions creates consistent results."

— CHRISTINE KANE

Staying true to the bedtime routine means having to listen to those cries without giving in to the urge to take your baby back into your arms to comfort them. Having been through this myself, I know how tough this can be for you to overcome. In this chapter, I'll share with you some tips that have helped me stay consistent with the goals of sleep training despite these challenges.

Recognizing When Your Baby Is Ready to Sleep

Your little one won't be able to say that they want to go to sleep, but various behavioral signs can tell you if they are feeling tired enough to fall asleep. Learning how to do spot them is easier said than done, however.

Many new parents tend to overlook these behavioral cues, especially the subtler ones such as rubbing the eyes or nose. Some misinterpret the cues as meaning something different, like hunger or pain. It can also go the other way, where a distress signal is mistaken as a sleep cue.

As a result, the schedule for the baby's sleep can be messed up. For example, Ben assumed that fussiness was always a sign that Max, his 3-month-old baby, wanted to sleep. Because of this, he ended up trying to put his baby to bed earlier than necessary. The bedtime routine did not work in winding down Max to a drowsy state. Instead, his baby continued to cry and be fussy no matter what he did.

In another instance, Ben noticed that Max tended to suck his thumb when he was feeling hungry. However, what he had failed to notice was that his baby also did this behavior whenever he felt tired. This mistake caused Max to become overtired. You might be thinking that fatigue would make it faster for babies to fall asleep, but on the contrary, being in this overtired state is quite distressful for infants so they actually find it even harder to go to sleep.

As you see, the optimal timing for putting your baby to sleep depends largely on how observant you are of their sleeping habits and behavioral cues. This becomes an even bigger challenge for those who are taking care of babies who are younger than 4 months old, who are likely not following any sort of pattern yet.

Fortunately, experts have noted the common sleep cues that babies from different age groups have been known to exhibit. Let's go over each of them so that you can better decide if it is time for your little one to go to sleep, and what would likely happen if you failed to notice the signs of tiredness.

A. Newborn to 3 Months Old

Babies at the younger end of the spectrum are mostly governed by their instincts. They also have minimal control over the movements of their limbs, so their actions are likely reflexive rather than deliberate. Because of this, the signs of tiredness that may be observed in this age group differ from the others.

Some of these signs are easy to spot. For example, when Max was just born, he would become fussy if he felt tired. This fussiness would then lead to whining and crying, and if his parents still failed to pay attention at that point, his cries would escalate to full-on screaming.

My second baby, Anne, had a different set of tired-ness-related behaviors. First, I would notice her glazed stare, which she would shift away from mine whenever I tried to look back. If that was not enough, she would turn her head away and then arch her back. This behavioral pattern is not usually seen among older babies, nor is it something that parents would automatically associate with tiredness or sleepiness. Other examples of similar signs that may escape your attention are:

- Sucking or needing to be fed to feel comfort
- Grimaced facial expression
- Clenched fists
- Jerky arms and legs
- Pulling the knees up to the chest

As you may have noticed, some of these signs may be linked to other states, such as hunger, pain, or distress due to overstimulation. What you can do to be certain that the behaviors you are seeing are indi-cating tiredness is to go through their probable causes and eliminate the ones that do not apply in the context of the situation.

For instance, to eliminate hunger from the list, think about the last time your baby has been fed. Has it been long enough for your little one to feel hungry again? Younger babies are also in the oral stage of their development. Therefore, wanting to be fed or sucking on their thumb may be caused by a wide variety of reasons other than hunger, like their need for comfort, rest, or relief.

If your baby has a seemingly painful look on his face, check him all over for injuries or illness. Sometimes, babies will also curl into a fetal position when they feel stomach pain. However, this would likely mean something else if your baby is not exhibiting the other common symptoms, such as diarrhea, vomiting, or lack of appetite.

Another variable that influences how babies in this age group exhibit tiredness is their general temperament. Even-tempered babies, for example, tend to fall asleep without much struggle from them or their parents. Those who are slow to warm up also take a long time before their fussiness escalates to crying or screaming.

On the other hand, babies with low tolerance points when it comes to having their needs met will become upset quicker if their parents fail to immediately notice their signs of tiredness.

Regardless of their temperament, babies who have reached the point of overtiredness have a hard time falling asleep. It can seem like they are resisting their drowsiness, or as if something is keeping them from sleep.

Moreover, infants in this age group tend to become overstimulated quickly. Babies who fall into this state will not respond well to their usual sleep aids, like being rocked or nursed to sleep.

Coupled with overstimulation, overtiredness can turn your bedtime routine into a tough challenge that can be upsetting and distressful for both you and your baby. If none of your sleep-inducing strategies have worked, sleep will eventually come to your baby once they have completely exhausted themselves.

B. 3 to 12 Months Old

By their third month of age, babies usually start to have more control over their limb movements. The jerky movements of their arms and legs will occur less frequently. If you recall, this is one of the signs of tiredness exhibited by younger babies.

Given their increased motor control, other signs that you should pay attention to include the following:

- Rubbing their hands against their eyes or nose
- Pulling their ears
- Pulling their hair

Yawning as a sign of tiredness is also typically observed among babies in this age group.

Some tiredness-related behavioral patterns are still found in this age group. For example, many infants of this age will still fuss and whine whenever they feel tired. This fussiness can escalate to crying and screaming if they have not been put to sleep.

The great thing is parents will find it easier to prevent their babies from suffering from overtiredness. At this point in development, infants will start developing relatively stable sleeping and eating patterns. This makes this period the optimal time for parents to get involved through various parenting strategies such as sleep training.

Don't be too complacent though. Some parents still overlook the signs of tiredness for various reasons, such as their baby's delicate temperament. Others might have too much on their plate, especially since some parents go back to work within this period.

Whatever the case may be, overtiredness among babies in this age group can be exhibited through heightened clinginess to their parents. Aside from wanting to be held all the time, an overtired baby will not be satisfied unless they are being rocked in your arms, or you are walking around while holding them.

When taken to the extreme, overtiredness can be quite distressful for everyone involved. The baby may start screaming, banging their head, biting, hitting anything or anyone within reach, or arching their back. If you try to console them using toys, they will just throw them away. Similarly, they will throw food and refuse to eat or drink anything.

Putting the baby down in their crib is not a good option either. They will just cry even harder. This highly distressful situation usually ends when the baby has no more energy left, leaving them no other option but to sleep.

C. Over 12 Months Old

Past their twelfth month of age, most babies become more of a handful to raise. They can now satisfy their natural curiosity about the world and people around them as they continue to practice walking and running around.

As they explore more of their surroundings, these babies will start feeling the need to be more independent from their parents. After all, those people are just going to put them to sleep even when they don't want to go.

Signs of tiredness for babies of this age are similar to the ones who are 3 to 12 months old. However, since they are more capable of doing things on their own, you may also notice a loss of body and arm coordination. As a result, your tired baby will likely spill their drink more than usual, bump into things as they play around, or even fall over when they walk.

Expect your baby to resist your attempts to follow the bedtime routine. If you have not sleep-trained them yet, it may be harder for you to convince them to cooperate with you, even if they are already feeling tired.

Given this, you should be mindful of the signs that your baby is already overtired. The tricky part is that this varies depending on their temperament. Some tend to display defiance by biting, hitting, screaming, or refusing to listen to instructions. Tantrums caused by things that don't usually upset them may also occur.

Others become hyperactive instead. Unlike adults who feel sluggish when they are overtired, these babies will suddenly get another burst of energy. Though you might be tempted to just leave them be until they tire themselves out, refrain from doing so since their sleep that night would be anything but restful. It would also keep them from staying consistent with their bedtime routine.

Make the effort to learn about your baby's signs of tiredness. By doing this, you will know when you should lay your baby down in their crib and bid goodnight. Remember, one of the rules of a good and healthy bedtime routine is letting your little one fall asleep on their own.

Knowing what to anticipate and how to interpret sleep cues will minimize the chances of overtiredness ruining the progress you have made. You will learn more about how to better handle an overtired baby in Chapter 5 of this book.

Keeping Yourself from Feeling Exhausted

According to Dr. Craig Canapari (2021), inconsistency is one of the biggest problems that he has observed among the parents who have consulted him at his sleep clinic. Various factors can lead to inconsistency, but exhaustion is a commonly given reason by parents who failed to carry out their babies' bedtime routine every night.

Aside from the higher probability of falling asleep in their child's bedroom, exhausted parents are likely not in the right mood for a gentle and soothing bedtime routine with their babies. They may also miss certain details that could be disruptive to the routine. In most cases, many will also be tempted to skip some parts of the routine, thus preventing their babies from completing their sleep training successfully.

It's understandable—after all, most parents have a lot of other things going on in their personal life, work, and other areas of responsibility. However, do not waste your time and effort, as well as your baby's progress in sleep training when you can do something about this issue.

Something to Think About...

Which of these sleep cues does your baby tend to exhibit?

Here's what you can do to keep your tiredness to a manageable level:

Tip #1: Pick a good starting date.

Sleep experts do not recommend beginning the training during certain periods, such as:

- Before moving out of a house
- Before going on a vacation
- Before a major surgery for any of the parents or immediate family members
- Before the birth of a new child in the family
- While your baby is teething
- While traveling with your baby

Many parents recommend starting on a Friday night so that the worst parts of the sleep training fall on a weekend, where people usually have more control over their time. If it's an option for you, consider taking some time off from work, too. By doing that you would be able to focus more on sleep training your baby, while also getting enough time to rest yourself.

"A perfect example of minority rule is a baby in the house."

— MILWAUKEE JOURNAL

Tip #2: Avoid having too much on your plate.

Other than a good starting date, you also should cancel or adjust certain activities that you normally do. While sleep training your baby, try your best to avoid going out all day to run errands or for late-night social activities.

Tip #3: Figure out why you are so tired.

Take the time to reflect on the probable factors that may be causing your exhaustion aside from sleep training. Is it work-related? Are you having other family issues that are draining your energy? Have you accepted too many obligations all at once?

For a more objective analysis, list your daily activities and use that as your guide in evaluating which areas of your life are contributing to your exhaustion. By pinpointing them, you will be able to decide what to do next, and how you can have more energy left for sleep training your baby.

Tip #4: Get others involved.

While you might want to be with your baby at every step of their sleep training, there are times when you should let others take over. It may be your partner, other adult members of the family, or your baby's caretaker.

Just remember to familiarize them with your baby's preferences, bedtime routine, sleep cues, and feeding schedules. Inconsistency can also occur if your mother-in-law decides to follow a different set of standards and rules while she is "helping" you with sleep training.

Do note that your baby may respond differently depending on who will be with them during bedtime. However, sometimes relying on others may have less of an effect on their bedtime routine than being with you when you don't have the energy for it.

Another probable cause of exhaustion among parents during sleep training is the sound of their baby crying before or in the middle of their sleep. The next section tackles how this can cause inconsistency in your baby's sleep routine and what you should do about it.

To Comfort or Not to Comfort a Crying Baby

No matter what sleep training method you choose, expect your baby to shed some—or a lot of—tears, especially during the initial days. Since they are not yet able to verbalize their reaction toward these changes in their day-to-day routine, many babies will exhibit resistance in this way.

This reaction can be observed more often among babies who are 5 months old or older. At that point in their development, they have already formed some bedtime habits and sleep associations that will be affected by sleep training.

On the other hand, younger babies are more open to these changes. They will only know what you have taught them so far, so their crying episodes tend to be shorter or less frequent.

Crying at night usually happens when you put down your baby in the crib, but it can also occur if your baby suddenly wakes up in the middle of their sleep. Either way, resisting acting upon hearing this is hard for most parents.

What makes this even harder for some is the belief that crying is always a sign of distress among babies. As such, parents must respond right away to soothe their baby until the crying stops. This involves unsustainable behaviors like rocking the baby in your arms, feeding them even if it is not the right time yet, or giving in to what they want.

But is it bad to let your baby cry out and not do anything about it?

It depends on the situation.

If you are certain that your baby isn't ill, hurt, or in any mortal danger, then you can leave them in their rooms even if you see or hear them cry. Make sure your baby does not feel hungry or does not need to have their diaper changed since those could be causing their distress, too.

If none of these conditions are affecting your baby, then more likely than not, their cries are mere attempts to seek your attention. While they are upset to be left on their own, they can manage it eventually and stop their crying without your help.

Since one of your goals for sleep training your baby is to teach them how to self-soothe until they fall asleep on their own, below are some valuable tips that can help parents accomplish this:

Tip #1: Make them feel comfortable.

Some of the activities I suggested in Chapter 2 are effective in making babies feel comfortable before bed—for instance, feeding your baby, giving them a warm bath, and changing them into their pajamas.

Their surroundings play a critical part in this, too. Make sure that the temperature in their bedroom is nice and cool—somewhere between 68°F (20°C) and 72°F (22°C). Opt for soft lighting that can be dimmed as your baby nears the time to sleep. Consider soundproofing their bedroom as well, in case there is a chance that outside noises may startle your baby as they try to go to sleep.

Ensuring your baby's comfort will eliminate some factors that could be causing them distress and preventing them from falling asleep.

Tip # 2: Avoid creating new or relying on existing sleep associations.

Sleep associations are essentially shortcuts for parents to get their babies to fall asleep again. It's so tempting to fall back into rocking or nursing your baby in your arms, especially when they start crying at three in the morning.

However, sleep associations are also known as "sleep crutches" for a reason. They can be bad for both you and your baby. Being dependent on them means that every time your baby has to sleep, you would have to rock, nurse, or even sing to them. Since your baby may wake up multiple times in one night, you would also have to engage in the same activities over and over again.

It's tiring and unsustainable for parents and may lead to sleep deprivation after a while. Furthermore, your baby will likely cry longer and harder every time you do not have the energy or willpower to carry out their sleep crutches. To better understand sleep associations, the next chapter will discuss their impact on your baby's sleep, as well as ways to effectively phase them out.

Tip #3: Comfort your baby from outside their bedroom.

If your baby wakes up in the middle of their sleep, refrain from hurrying back inside their bedroom to comfort them in your arms until they fall asleep again. If it is not an emergency, it's best to give them the chance to soothe themselves.

To do this, set up a baby monitor in their bedroom, preferably one that has a camera function. Check your baby's well-being through this device when you hear them crying. Other than life-endangering situations, opt to either let them cry without your interference or try to comfort them from outside their bedroom.

As much as possible, avoid showing yourself to your baby while they are crying. Your presence may agitate them even more. If they are crying for attention, seeing you would just spur them on since it will teach them that crying is an effective means of getting what they want.

Rather than letting your child see you as a means of comfort, talk to them instead. The sound of your voice may be enough to calm down your baby, while also not being as intrusive as your physical presence.

Tip #4: Practice controlled comforting.

If you have adopted the gradual extinction strategy, controlled comforting may be a good way to teach your baby how to self-soothe. However, this is best suited for babies who are over 6 months old—

though it may take you longer if you apply this to toddlers.

How does it work?

Controlled comforting involves periodically checking on and soothing your baby throughout the night. The gentler pace, compared to CIO or Weissbluth methods, allows babies to get used to the idea of going to sleep on their own. It also allows them to figure out how to self-comfort well enough to go back to sleep without needing help from their parents.

I recommend going for the controlled comforting strategy on the second day of sleep training your baby. Through this, you and your baby will be able to remain consistent with the established bedtime routine, while also reducing the emotional and mental stress that crying could cause for both of you.

As a guide, follow the steps below to ensure that Day 2 of your baby's sleep training will be a success:

1. Go through the bedtime routine you established on Day 1 of sleep training. Don't skip or change an activity. Be mindful of the timing as well.

2. Lay your baby in their crib while they are still awake. Say something sweet and gentle to your little one. Keep it short—about a minute or two. Then, quietly leave their bedroom.

3. Listen to your baby from outside the bedroom. For about a minute or two, listen to check if your baby will cry. If all you can hear is the sound of whining or fussing, then just wait until your baby has settled without your help. You may leave once your baby is making no more sounds.

4. If you hear your baby crying, wait for a bit before heading back inside.

Remember to set the waiting time beforehand. I suggest waiting for five minutes, but depending on the temperament of your baby, it may be as brief as two minutes.

If you are going for a five-minute initial waiting time, the next time your baby cries, your waiting time must be increased up to 10 minutes. In the third instance, it may be a 12-minute waiting time.

Intervals can also be smaller. For example, you can follow a two-minute increment for each time your baby cries. Again, go for what would work best for you and your baby.

For longer timed intervals, you can go to other parts of your house instead of waiting the entire time outside your baby's room. For example, go to the kitchen and make yourself a cup of tea.

5. Head back inside your baby's bedroom.

If the waiting time has lapsed and your baby is still crying, you may go back to their side and offer them comfort. Remember though: Your goal is not to make them fall asleep again. Your baby just needs to stop crying and calm down.

As much as possible, avoid picking up your baby in your arms. Instead, opt for soft pats or gentle words. Aim to keep this interaction as brief as you can. In my experience, it didn't last for more than a minute.

Quick Tip!

Use the alarm function of your mobile device to keep track of the timed intervals. Remember to set it to vibrate mode only. though since the alarm sound may disrupt your baby's sleep.

6. Leave your baby's room again.

Once you are outside, listen and check for signs that your baby is either starting to wind down or crying again. If it's the latter, wait until your next timed interval has lapsed before repeating Step 5.

7. Continue doing the controlled comforting until your baby has fallen asleep.

If your baby wakes up again and cries before their supposed waking time, check to make sure they are feeling okay before attempting to comfort them. Here are some ideas of what you should do:

- Take a look at the room temperature to see if it's still within the ideal range.
- Gently touch your baby to see if they are feeling hot or cold.
- Look for any signs that they are feeling ill or unwell, such as coughing, chills, or short, rapid breaths.
- Make sure to check their diaper just to be sure that they don't need to be changed.

While it is advisable to push through the bedtime routine and the rest of your sleep training plan despite hearing your baby cry, remember to pay attention to their reactions and feelings. If it seems like they are becoming too distressed with your chosen method, I highly suggest seeking the guidance of a child development professional.

By Day 2 of their sleep training, your baby will start adapting to the changes in their routine, so be patient and remain strong in your conviction to improve your baby's sleep habits.

However, babies' tears are kryptonite for many parents. I've been through this several times—I know how powerful they can be in chipping away at my commitment to stay consistent. I'd like to be able to tell you that the whining and crying will stop by the third night, but the first three to four days of sleep training tend to be filled with tears. In the next chapter, I will show you what to expect on Day 3 of sleep training, and how you and your baby can get through it without breaking your consistency streak.

4

DAY 3: PREPARE FOR TEARS

Sleep training and crying babies seem to go hand in hand for many people. It's not exactly a wrong assumption, but it also oversimplifies why babies cry when parents attempt to sleep train them.

By now, I have repeatedly warned you about the intense crying episodes that normally occur during the second and third night of sleep training.

Many inexperienced parents assume that such nights are signs that the training is too upsetting for their babies. As a result, they believe that their chosen method isn't working at all. Giving up immediately seems to be the right course of action, but as you will learn in this chapter, there is more than meets the eye when a baby cries.

To help you get through Day 3 of sleep training your baby, we will discuss why babies cry so hard sometimes, as well as how you can harness the powerful influence of sleep associations on your baby's quality of sleep to better manage and reduce their crying episodes. By the end of this chapter, you will also learn what you should do if you hear your baby crying during sleep training.

Take Note!

The onset of extinction burst may vary depending on your chosen sleep training strategy as well as the temperament and sensitivity level of your baby. Those who follow extinction-based strategies experience them earlier than those who adapt gentler approaches.

Intense Crying and Sleep Training

Behavioral psychologists use the term "extinction burst" to describe the period where an individual who is trying to get rid of bad behavior will somehow behave even worse before improving for the better. In sleep training. this phenomenon can be observed early on.

On the first night of sleep training, most parents say that their babies cried when they left them in the bedroom. More often than not, their actual experiences weren't as bad as they were expecting.

However, by the second and third night, those same parents were shocked to see their babies not just crying but also screaming and jerking around in the crib. Some babies cried so hard that they threw up before succumbing to exhaustion and falling into a night of restless sleep. In certain cases, older babies even attempted to jump out of their crib, which could potentially cause injuries if they had landed badly.

At this point, parents who do not know any better would give up. Seeing their children act like this for more than an hour can easily dissolve their confidence about the effectiveness of sleep training.

On the other hand, those who are aware that their babies are likely going through an extinction burst would see these intense episodes as a sign that progress is being made. They understand that these negative reactions will subside soon, and improvements can be expected soon after.

Why do extinction bursts happen during sleep training though?

Since babies have limited means of communicating their needs and wants, crying serves as one of their ways to get their parents' attention. When parents try to placate and comfort their babies whenever they cry, this behavior will be reinforced. This means whenever they need or want something done, these babies will cry out.

In sleep training, parents are highly encouraged to refrain from acting upon the fussing and crying of their babies. On the first night, the little ones will likely not notice that things are changing in their normal routine.

However, by the second and third nights, many babies will realize that their regular crying is not enough anymore. They need to go louder and stronger to grab their parents' attention again. The sudden wailing, screaming, and resistance to fall asleep characterize this phase of extinction bursts during sleep training.

Yes, it is perfectly understandable you would have some second thoughts about pushing forward. Rest assured that extinction bursts are normal when it comes to behavioral change. You are one step closer to your goal!

In general, the effects of extinction burst subside by Day 4 or Day 5 of sleep training. That's something to look forward to, right? However, you still must go through the dreaded Day 3. Based on the gradual extinction strategy, here's an outline of my recommendations to get you through this night.

1. Perform the established bedtime routine for your baby.

This should be the same one you did on Day 1 and Day 2. This will ensure they adapt the new and healthier routine through consistency.

2. Put your baby in the crib, then leave the room.

Remember, you are teaching them to self-soothe. Even if they tend to fuss and cry when you leave them on their own, let them be.

3. If you hear your baby cry, wait for 10 minutes before returning to their bedroom.

This is what differentiates this method from other extinction-based strategies, such as CIO. You are not leaving your child for the rest of the night. You just have to wait for 10 to 15 minutes outside your baby's room, and then you may head back inside to reassure them of your presence.

Why should you wait though?

Studies show that immediately responding to the cries of a baby will make it harder for you to leave them again (Gradisar et al, 2016). You will notice that if you do this, your little one will start crying again as soon as you put them back in the crib or when you leave their room.

4. Adjust the waiting time to 12 minutes if your baby cries again after the first instance.

If your baby cries more than two times that night, increase the succeeding waiting times to 15 minutes. Keep in mind that for each return to your baby's bedroom, your goal is not to stop their crying or to get them back to sleep. Instead, reassure them that they are fine and that you are nearby if they need you.

One of the critical goals during Day 3 is to refrain from relying on your baby's bad sleep associations, even if you hear them crying in the middle of the night. Bad sleep associations can be effective in making babies stop crying and guiding them back to sleep. However, they are bad for a reason—as you will learn in the next section.

Let your baby learn how to soothe themselves without your help, even if it's heartbreaking for you to hear them fuss and cry. Otherwise, you will only reinforce their bad sleep associations and prevent them from embracing the good ones that you want to teach your baby.

Sleep Associations: Good or Bad?

We have talked about sleep associations for the past few chapters of this book. If you recall, sleep associations can be anything that could induce sleep. Everyone has them—knowingly or unknowingly.

By now, you know that sleep training your baby involves weaning them off of their bad sleep associations and replacing those with good ones. But what exactly makes a sleep association good or bad for your baby?

Sleep associations of babies become either good or bad depending on who is performing them. Good sleep associations are sleep-related actions that can be carried out by your baby without any help from others. For example:

- Hitting the crib mattress with their hands or feet

- Holding, rubbing, or chewing a soft blanket or toy
- Humming or singing to themselves
- Lifting their knees into a fetal position
- Rocking themselves from side to side

On the other hand, those that require your help or intervention are considered bad sleep associations. Why? It's not the action itself that is negative or ineffective, it is the fact that someone else needs to be involved just so your baby can fall asleep. Here are some examples of common bad sleep associations that you may be doing for your baby:

- Bouncing, rocking, or swinging in your arms
- Holding your baby's hand
- Nursing or bottle-feeding to sleep
- Pushing them around in a stroller or driving them around in your car until they fall asleep
- Singing a lullaby to your baby
- Sleeping beside—or even inside—the crib

A bad sleep association can be something as bond-strengthening as nursing your baby to sleep, or as effective as rocking them in your arms. They can be used as shortcuts during bedtime, but what happens when no one else is there to do them for your baby?

What if your baby wakes up in the middle of the night, and they can't fall back to sleep unless you nurse or rock them again? Exhausted parents who have to get up at 3 a.m. just to make their babies stop crying and put them back to sleep know exactly how the rest of this goes.

Did you know that...

Baby pacifiers fall somewhere in between good and bad sleep associations? While sucking on them can be done by your baby without needing your help, it can be unsustainable too if you have to go back to your baby's room just so you can reinsert the pacifier into their mouths every time they wake up at night.

In comparison, babies with good sleep associations are less likely to cry at night even if their sleep is suddenly interrupted. They know how to soothe themselves through their learned sleep associations. As a result, you and your baby will not suffer the consequences brought about by bad sleeping habits that could have been phased out during sleep training.

Good sleep associations can be something external, too. By setting up an optimal sleeping area for your baby, you are teaching them to associate those conditions with sleep—for instance, the sound from a white noise machine, the dimness of the room due to blackout shades, and the comfort brought about by being in a room that is neither too hot nor too cold.

Soft blankets or toys can be part of a good sleep association if you let your baby sleep while holding on to them. Just be extra careful in selecting and placing the blanket or toy in their crib. Make sure that your baby could easily remove it from their face or nose in case it hinders their breathing.

Effects of Sleep Associations

Addressing your baby's sleep associations have short-term and long-term impacts on their health and development.

Short-term effects can be observed in three aspects: how easy it is for your baby to fall asleep, how long your baby can stay asleep, and how prone your baby is to overtiredness.

Falling Asleep

Babies need the help of their parents or caregivers to go to sleep—from being carried to bed and setting up the right bedroom condition to establishing sleeping routines. Your level of involvement will influence the kind of sleep associations that your baby will develop. Whether good or bad, they are going to look for them whenever you try to put them to sleep.

If your baby's sleep associations have been carried out, then you may expect them to fall asleep quickly and with minimal or no tears at all. However, if they have been withheld, your baby will fuss, whine, or cry in an attempt to push you into giving them what they want.

Though you might want to just rely on these sleep associations to put your baby to sleep, remember that you should let your baby keep only the ones that they can do on their own. If you allow your baby to become dependent on sleep associations that require the participation of other people, you will be putting them at risk of having trouble falling asleep.

Staying Asleep

Sleep associations that are relatively noticeable, such as background music or rocking your baby while holding them, can cause your baby to wake up too soon. During the deep parts of their sleep cycle, your baby will likely not notice if you have put them down in their crib.

However, once they enter the lighter parts, there is a chance that they will notice the lack of music or rocking motion. If they notice, their sleep will be interrupted. Depending on how much sleep they have gotten at that point, your baby can either wake up feeling well-rested or cranky.

Babies who can self-soothe and have good sleep associations can return to sleep without much of a fuss. On the other hand, those with bad ones will find it hard to go back to sleep unless someone helps them carry out their sleep associations.

Overtiredness

Babies who depend on bad sleep associations are more at risk of overtiredness compared to those with good sleep associations. Whether these associations affect their ability to fall asleep quickly or their capacity to stay asleep, overtiredness tends to be a consequence of ignoring this issue.

As explained in the previous chapter of this book, an overtired baby is not able to sleep no matter how much they need to rest. Instead, they are going to fuss, scream, or cry to point of physical exhaustion. By then, they will fall asleep with or without the presence of their sleep association.

Waiting for your child to get to that point can only bring negative effects to their health and development. Imagine how much more harm this could cause if you let this problem recur repeatedly for a long time.

Long-term effects of sleep associations can be observed once babies enter the childhood phase of their development. A longitudinal study conducted among pre-school children and their parents highlighted how sleeping problems that originated in early childhood persisted even when the children were already between ages 29 and 40 months (Simard et al, 2008). Their poor sleep associations continued to be part of their regular sleeping routine, and so they continued to have difficulties in falling and staying asleep throughout the night.

If such sleep problems remain unaddressed, the problem won't be just one sleepless night after another. Several long-term studies have been conducted over the years to ascertain the true impact of inadequate sleep and poor sleep quality on one's development and wellness. For example, a British study by Reilly et al (2005) showed that the participating children who frequently got fewer than 10.5 hours of sleep per day had a 45% probability of becoming obese by age seven.

Given the probable effects of sleep associations on you and your baby, you have the option to just let them be—if you believe that they are just minor ones that do not significantly hamper their sleeping routine—or to make some necessary changes to improve their current sleep associations.

Aside from basing your decision on who currently carries out your babies sleep associations, you must consider the following three factors:

A. Awareness of Surroundings

The older your baby is, the more aware they are of what's happening around them. Conversely, those who are younger are less aware, thus allowing them to remain asleep even if you stop performing their sleep associations or change their sleeping positions into a more comfortable one.

Quick Tip!

Don't worry about sleep associations if your baby is 3 months old or younger. They are too young to sleep on their own so it's fine if you rely on some sleep associations like singing to them or holding their hands as they fall asleep.

Start addressing your baby's sleep associations by the time they are around 4 to 6 months old. Your goals are to phase out any bad sleep associations that they have formed so far and to guide them into learning new ones that could help them self-soothe.

This period, however, changes by the time babies reach their fourth month. Around this time, their mental growth gets a burst of development. They become more and more aware of the changes that occur around them while they are conscious and during the lighter parts of the sleep cycle. Because of this, many babies go through the so-called "4-month sleep regression," where their waking hours are greater than their sleep hours. Further discussion about sleep regression will be covered in the next chapter.

If your baby has become sensitive to changes in their environment, consider it as a signal that you should start working on improving their sleep associations. They are going to be harder to put to sleep, and they are more prone to waking up in the middle of sleep. Having good sleep associations will help them get through these issues with fewer tears.

Fortunately, at this stage of their development, sleep training is an optimal solution that could provide long-lasting effects on the length and quality of your baby's sleep. I highly suggest guiding your baby into developing good sleep associations.

B. Temperament

Your baby's temperament also influences how sensitive they are to changes. Those who are on the carefree end of the spectrum tend to have better and longer sleep. Even if they go through a period of sleep regression, the changes will likely not bother them to the point of disrupting their normal sleep cycle. Yes, they may still form bad sleep associations, but these babies are more cooperative when it comes to their parents' attempts to phase those habits out of their daily routine.

On the other hand, sensitive infants are more likely to suffer from sleepless nights than their more easy-going counterparts. The higher their level of sensitivity, the greater the risk of developing sleep-related problems, such as overtiredness and sleep deprivation.

Guiding sensitive babies into forgetting their learned sleep associations can be tough, but not impossible. They will notice what you are attempting to do and react more intensely, such as more whining, crying, and screaming. However, giving up on sleep training sensitive babies just because of its difficulty will leave them suffering from sleep problems that could snowball into even bigger health and developmental issues later on.

According to Benoit (2004), roughly 55% of infants belong to the sensitive end of the spectrum. That means your baby has a slightly higher chance of being sensitive to changes, but it also means that you are not alone when it comes to sleep training a sensitive baby. Getting rid of their bad sleep associations is a perfectly achievable goal for any parent to pursue.

C. Existing Sleep Associations

Your baby's response toward your attempt to improve their sleeping routine will also depend on the type and quantity of sleep associations they currently have. Take for example the differences between my firstborn, Alex, and youngest child, Kate.

When Alex was only 3 months old, I used to put him to sleep by swinging him in my arms while he sucked on his pacifier. Once he fell asleep, I would lay him down in his crib and leave.

While he was in deep sleep, the changes in his sleeping position did not bother him at all. However, I noticed that he would suddenly wake up crying in the middle of the night as if sensing that I was no longer holding him and that there was no swinging motion anymore. It didn't help that his pacifier would usually fall out of his mouth during his sleep.

In comparison, Kate was a better sleeper at around the same age. This might be because I had already experienced and learned how sleep associations could affect my child's sleep. Rather than doing the same things I did for Alex's bedtime routine, I made it a point to tuck Kate in for the night just before she fell asleep.

Yes, Kate still fussed when I refrained from touching her as a way to get her to sleep, and even when she woke up in the middle of the night my soft pats were just gestures of reassurance and comfort—not my means to put her back to sleep.

Other than the type of sleep associations Alex and Kate had as babies, Alex relied on more sleep crutches than his sister. Because of this, the changes in his sleeping conditions were more significant than Kate's. Therefore, even if your baby is not particularly sensitive, they will likely notice and react if you make a lot of changes in how they usually go to sleep.

However, regardless of whether your baby is more like either Alex or Kate, you should pay careful attention to the other two factors when deciding about your next course of action about their sleep associations. Yes, your little one might not be fussy now, but once they have entered their period of sleep regression, their easygoing temperament might not be enough to keep them from spending more time awake than asleep.

Observe your baby based on these three factors and evaluate how much help your baby needs when it comes to dealing with their sleep associations. If your baby is anything like Kate, then you only have to do a few adjustments to remove their bad sleep associations. This means you can focus more on developing better sleep associations instead.

On the other hand, if your little one depends on several bad sleep associations, your next goal should be to help your baby unlearn those bad sleeping habits and then redirect them into developing good ones.

Unlearning Bad Sleep Associations and Developing Good Sleep Associations

---

"I like changing diapers. There's a beginning, middle, and an end, so I feel accomplished. When the baby is crying and you can't communicate with it, then I'm frustrated. At least with the diaper, I know that it started dirty and now it's clean."

— SETH MEYERS

Sleep training can be an effective way to address your baby's sleep associations. However, to effectively avoid or remove a sleep association, you must first learn how they are formed in the first place.

Babies learn through regular repetition. If something has been done repeatedly, an association will be formed in their brains, thus helping them make connections between actions and their experiences.

Studies show that babies can start learning sleep associations within a few days or weeks of birth. You might not be aware of it, but there's a high chance that you have been teaching your infant a sleep association this whole time.

For example, you might have a habit of gently stroking your newborn baby's tummy until she falls asleep. If you continually stroke her tummy every time she has to sleep, she will learn to associate tummy stroking with sleeping. This will be part of her bedtime preferences, and if she also happens to be a sensitive baby, there will be no other way to get her to sleep without her tummy being gently stroked.

Your baby will develop this connection between stroking and sleeping whether you want them to or not. Don't feel bad though because, as explained earlier, most younger babies need sleep associations, and you can start phasing out the bad ones that have formed once you start sleep training them.

Since sleep associations are formed through consistency, they can also be removed in the same manner. Once you have decided to stop doing it, be strong and stay committed to your goal. For instance, once I started sleep training Alex in his fourth month, I refrained from swinging him in my arms before bed.

Sounds simple enough, right?

The tough part is facing the reactions of your baby. Expect a lot of whining and crying as your baby tries to adjust to the changes in their sleeping routine and conditions.

The great thing about babies is that most of them seem to be naturals at learning how to self-soothe. When Alex realized that I would not be holding and swinging him to sleep despite his tears and screams, he began to move slightly from side to side, as if he was trying to mimic the swinging motion I used to do for him. Since that was something that he could do without my help, I recognized it as a good sleep association that Alex should keep.

Developing other good sleep associations can also be done through consistency. Choose a sleep training method that will work for you and your baby, and then incorporate good sleep associations as a part of your planned bedtime routine for your baby. Be consistent night after night to strengthen the connection between those sleep associations and sleeping.

Again, your baby might resist the changes you are bringing into their routine. Normally, this would last for only a few days before they embrace the new sleep associations.

However, those few days can be hellish, not just for your baby, but also for you. It may be a serious test of your ability to stay consistent with the goals of sleep training your baby. To help parents go through such nights, below are some excellent tips that could work for you too:

Tip #1: Calm down by doing your preferred "time-out" techniques.

Perform self-calming techniques that help you maintain your level-headedness. Some parents opt for breathing techniques, while others prefer to walk around the house for a few minutes. Feel free to do what works for you, as long as it does not interfere with sleep training your baby.

Tip #2: Say some positive affirmations to yourself.

These may be full sentences or phrases as long as the words can give you the motivation to push through despite how tough the situation is. Positive affirmations can also help you stay focused on what matters and remind you about why you are doing this in the first place.

Let me share some of the positive affirmations that I have said to myself while sleep training my children:

- "Breathe in and breathe out—everything is going to be fine."
- "This is perfectly normal, and all will be well in the end."
- "I am focused and calm. My baby is fine and healthy."
- "I can keep going for my baby and my family."

Tip #3: Learn the different kinds of cries that your child has.

This bears great importance especially for babies who have not yet learned how to speak. Sometimes, their cries can be a signal for pain, illness, and incredible distress. Pay attention to how your baby is crying—the pitch, volume, incessantness, and if you have a baby monitor trained on them, check if your baby looks rigid, too. Learn to differentiate their cries so that you can act accordingly when the time comes.

Tip #4: Seek the help of others.

You don't have to be on top of everything for every single night of your baby's sleep training. If you are not in the right mood or mindset for it, consider tapping others to take over in the meantime. You will find it extra hard to resist your child's tears if you are feeling down or unwell yourself. Just make sure that whoever will be stepping in for you is also well-oriented about why and how you are sleep training your baby.

While I can't completely guarantee that these tips will also be effective for you—after all, everyone faces different circumstances in life—I can attest that they helped me immensely during the second and third days of sleep training. I do hope that what you have learned in this chapter will prepare you well enough to face and overcome the most challenging parts of this endeavor.

After learning how to properly manage the tearful nights of sleep training, you can now focus more on guiding your baby into developing healthy sleep patterns. The next chapter will show you how you can start doing this on the fourth and fifth days of your baby's sleep training.

5

DAYS 4 AND 5: ENCOURAGE HEALTHY SLEEP PATTERNS

At this point of sleep training, your baby will likely fuss and cry less than they did for the past few days. They are starting to get accustomed to the new routine, so what you need to do is stay consistent with what you have been doing so far.

Rather than improving the routine by adding or removing bedtime activities, you should gradually increase the waiting time whenever you hear your child cry or suddenly wake up in the middle of the night. This way, you will give them more opportunities to learn how to self-soothe and go back to sleep on their own.

The suggested activity outlines for Days 4 and 5 are almost the same as the ones you have been following for the previous days: Put your baby down while they are drowsy—not fully asleep—and then say your goodnights and reassuring words, before finally leaving their bedroom quietly.

Here's where the differences come in. During Days 4 and Day 5, wait for 12 minutes outside your baby's bedroom if you hear them screaming and crying when you leave them on their own. Once the predetermined time has lapsed, head back inside, and try to briefly reassure them once more with your presence and gentle words.

Afterward, leave the bedroom again, and see if your baby will either cry again or fall asleep. If your baby starts crying again, increase the waiting time to 15 minutes. Repeat what you did earlier once you have held yourself back long enough.

"Despite having a million things to do, it is very difficult to look away from my sleeping baby. She is like a magnet!"

— MARIA JOSE OVALLE

There's a chance that your baby will still refuse to sleep. For all succeeding times after your second return to your baby's room, increase your waiting time to 17 minutes.

If you find yourself having trouble waiting this long, go back to the tips in the previous chapter, and do whatever will keep you from interfering with your baby's learning and adjustment process.

You might wonder by now how can you tell if what you have been doing is helping your baby to sleep better. After all, you have just experienced multiple nights that were likely filled with your baby's screaming and crying during bedtime.

One good way to determine the progress of your baby's sleep training is by observing their sleep patterns. Having a healthy sleep pattern is essential for babies to grow and develop well. This can be established through sleep training, but some factors —such as sleep regression and overtiredness—can keep your baby from having restful sleep.

That's why, for this chapter, I'll explain the healthy sleep pattern that your baby must adopt, as well as the ways to overcome the challenges that you and your baby might face along the way.

What Are Sleep Patterns?

Everyone has an internal biological clock that signals different bodily functions and conditions, such as hunger, excretion, and sleep, throughout the day. Babies have them too, but their clocks are still developing and prone to being influenced by various factors. As such, you can set and reset their patterns according to what would be optimal for their health and growth.

Since you are sleep training your baby, it's the optimal time to promote healthy sleep patterns. But first, what are sleep patterns?

Sleep patterns refer to the repetition of sleep cycles that occur throughout the night. When your baby is asleep, their body and mind aren't in just one constant state that changes only when they wake up.

Instead, regular sleep consists of five distinct stages, where a brief moment of wakefulness separates the current stage from the next. This occurs so fleetingly that barely anyone notices or remembers it happening during their sleep.

Each sleep cycle lasts for different durations depending on the person's age:

- Newborn: 20 to 40 minutes
- Babies to toddlers: 30 to 60 minutes
- Children: 40 to 90 minutes
- Adults: about 90 minutes

Given these, your baby may repeat a sleep cycle seven to nine times each night. During their nap, this repetition is far less at one to three times only for each naptime.

Let's go over the five stages of sleep that babies go through for each sleep cycle to better understand why their natural progression must be maintained.

Stage 1

Duration: About 5 to 10 minutes

This begins when your baby feels drowsy—that's why you must put them down in the crib at this time. Otherwise, you risk disrupting this stage when it has just begun. If you do put them down, your baby would likely fall into a light sleep in a matter of a few minutes.

Infants' eyelids will droop closed as their eyes roll upward. Some babies open and close their mouths too, while their breathing evens out.

Though your baby has officially entered the sleep cycle, they are still easy to wake up at this stage, so be careful not to touch or move them around.

Stage 2

Duration: Up to 20 minutes

During this entire period, your baby is in a light sleep state. You may hear them making some grunting noises and some babies tend to smile. Twitching and jerking limbs usually happen during this stage as well.

Again, your baby's sleep can easily be disrupted if they become startled by movements or sudden, loud noises. If they are woken up prematurely, expect them to fuss or cry for some time.

Stage 3 and Stage 4

These two stages of sleep closely resemble one another except for their respective depths. Simply speaking, your baby will be in a deeper sleep in Stage 4 compared to Stage 3.

To know whether your little one has reached this point, observe their breathing first. It should be slow but regularly paced. This indicates that their body and mind are both in a relaxed state. There is no twitching or jerking of arms or legs, and their facial expression is void of any emotion.

Babies in either Stage 3 or Stage 4 can be very hard to wake up. If there is a sudden movement or loud sound nearby, their reactions will be slower than usual. Often, babies fall right back to sleep after being prematurely woken up, unlike in the previous stages of sleep.

Stage 5

Duration: Varied (About 50% of sleeping time among babies and children, and about 20% among adults)

Of the five stages of a sleep cycle, this is the only one that involves Rapid Eye Movement (REM), which indicates a state where numerous brain activities occur during sleep.

Among those activities, the most important one is the release of hormones that are responsible for healing and growth. Since the body is at rest, it is the best time for the body to do repair work in different parts of the body. Babies and children get the extra benefit of getting a boost in their growth rate, too.

To determine whether your baby has already reached Stage 5 of their sleep cycle, pay attention to the following signs:

- Discernible movements of the eyeballs even when the eyelids are closed
- Increased heart rate
- Rapid and erratic breathing
- Twitching movements in the face, fingers, and legs

Take note that individuals who are in Stage 5 are experiencing light sleep, so this can be easy to disrupt as well. Because of what happens during REM sleep, it's incredibly important to completely pass through this stage uninterrupted, especially for babies.

Many inexperienced parents misinterpret the signs above as indications that their babies are about to wake up. As a result, some would pick up and hold their babies in their arms. Since the babies in this stage are in the lighter parts of their sleep, there is a high chance that they will be woken up prematurely. This hampers the internal body activities that occur during REM sleep, thus preventing babies from fully reaping their benefits.

Aside from failing to recognize the signs, the natural progression of sleep cycles can be negatively affected by other factors as well, such as:

- Being deprived of sleep
- Suffering from high levels of stress
- Experiencing frequent changes in their surroundings or schedules for sleeping and feeding

The challenges brought on from these three factors can manifest in various forms. Two of the most common challenges faced by parents and their babies are sleep regression and overtiredness. When these remain unaddressed for a significant amount of time, they can prevent your baby from developing healthy sleep patterns. Let's next discuss how you can manage and overcome these challenges while sleep training your baby.

"Sometimes going to bed feels like the highlight of my day. Ironically, to my children, bedtime is a punishment that violates their basic rights as human beings."

— JIM GAFFIGAN

Challenge #1: Sleep Regression

Upon finishing the newborn phase of their development, most babies won't need as much sleep as they did before. Previously, they needed about 16 to 17 hours of sleep per day. This will decrease to about 12 to 15 hours, which means longer waking hours during the day and more sleeping hours at night.

However, some babies go through sleep regression instead. This can go on for 2 to 4 weeks—though there are cases where it has lasted for up to 6 weeks.

During this period, the baby suddenly regresses to the sleeping habits of a newborn. Falling asleep becomes more troublesome again since their fussiness and crankiness seem to be heightened. They will wake up more frequently at night, screaming and crying for their parents. Meanwhile, during the day, napping starts to become a struggle again.

Why does this happen?

According to sleep experts, babies go through sleep regression due to various factors that may cause them discomfort, anxiety, or restlessness. For example, babies who are experiencing a growth spurt tend to feel hungry more often. As such, they wake up more frequently in the middle of the night to feed, as if they are newborns again. Other probable causes include:

- Pain due to the growth of baby teeth
- Excitement and exhaustion during significant developmental milestones, like crawling and walking
- Adjustment to a new environment or people while traveling
- Illness or injuries

Given these causes, sleep regression can happen at any point after your baby has exited the newborn phase of their development. Your baby may also go through it more than once. To help you better recognize its signs, here's a quick rundown of how sleep regression occurs at different ages:

3 to 4 Months

Many babies within this age range experience sleep regression because of the following reasons:

- Their baby teeth are starting to grow.
- They are about to have their first growth spurt.
- Their body control and motor skills have developed well enough for them to roll over for the first time.

The signs of sleep regression will persist and peak for about two to three weeks. Afterward, some babies will naturally go back to sleeping more at night without needing any intervention from their parents. Others, however, may need to have some of their existing sleep habits—especially the ones that involve bad sleep associations—to be changed through sleep training.

6 Months

At this point, a lot of babies get another growth spurt. If you started sleep training them before, then your baby can go back to sleep on their own, or with some reassurance from you through gentle words and soft touches. However, if you have not yet done so, this would be another good time to start sleep training your baby.

8 to 10 Months

Sleep regression occurs for babies in this age range because of either their new abilities or separation anxiety. At this point in their development, babies can explore more of their surroundings since many of them begin to crawl and stand on their own.

Did you know that...

Separation anxiety is a normal part of a baby's growth and development. Don't treat it in the same way as you do with the anxiety disorders that teens and adults may have. Learn more about separation anxiety in babies in the next chapter.

Not all developments are as exciting as this. In terms of mental abilities, these babies are more capable of noticing the lack of their parent's presence, especially during bedtime. This causes them to feel more anxious at the thought of being left alone in their crib, thus making them crave reassurance from their parents in the middle of the night.

12 Months

At this point, babies who undergo sleep regression also experienced it when they were 8 to 10 months old. As a result, this challenging period may pass quicker—typically no more than three weeks—than the previous ones because most babies have established a pretty good routine by this time.

Take Note!

Sleep regression is a natural phenomenon that happens because the sleeping patterns of babies are still evolving. It's a good sign that your baby is growing and developing normally. Though it may not happen to every baby, don't fret if your baby goes through it. It will pass; it is not a sickness that needs treatment, and you can survive this period with the help of the coping strategies and tips given in this chapter.

There are cases where sleep regression affects the naptimes of 11- to 12-month-old babies too. If this is happening with your baby, you will notice them trying to transition to only one nap per day—usually skipping the afternoon nap—or taking two shorter 45-minute naps instead.

The most likely cause of sleep regression for babies at this age is walking. A lot of babies take their first steps somewhere between ages 10 to 14 months. Though they cannot go on for long, these attempts to walk on their own tire them out fast. That's why some babies don't make the transition to one nap— they need to sleep some more to regain their energy.

18 Months

Your baby has turned into a toddler by this age. This can be particularly challenging because many toddlers relish their newfound independence. They can now walk and talk to some extent—an ability that also enables them to say no when they don't want to follow your instructions.

Teething pains will come into play here too. Toddlers are starting to grow their molars, so the discomfort brought about by this development will likely trigger another round of sleep regression for them.

You may also notice that your toddler is experiencing separation anxiety during naptime and bedtime. They can be genuinely distressed at the sight of you leaving them alone, but if you have sleep trained them by this point, your reassurances before stepping out of the bedroom may be enough to get them to self-soothe afterward and then sleep on their own.

24 Months

Toddlers experience a couple of important milestones during this age. Many parents begin potty training their kids at this time, while others move their toddlers out of the crib and into a child's bed. Some toddlers may also get a new sibling, which could affect them greatly, especially if they had been an only child up to this point.

At 24 months old, toddlers have longer waking hours, too. This adjustment might mess up their nap and sleep schedule, which could then trigger a sleep regression.

Having learned the probable causes of sleep regression, let's now discuss some techniques that can minimize their impact on your baby's sleep patterns:

Teething pain

To tell whether your baby is suffering from this, be on the lookout for the following signs: excessive drooling, increased fussiness when feeding, biting almost anything they could get their hands on, and general irritability.

It's best to consult your baby's pediatrician about the right ways to solve this one, especially if it seems to be a particularly painful case for your baby. You may provide comfort though—just refrain from moving them around or picking them up since it may only irritate them even more. Stick to gentle touches and words, and then leave the room to let them try to settle without any further interaction with you.

Illness

You know how irritating it is when you have a sore throat, congested nose, or a fever. Now imagine how your baby feels when they are sick and can't do much about it.

Of course, you need to seek the medical advice of your baby's pediatrician for such serious or sensitive health issues. Giving the right medication to your baby will not only speed up their healing and recovery, but will also hasten your baby's return to their bedtime routine.

Sometimes, babies will need extra attention from you when they are feeling ill. Yes, you can give them that but remember to go back to doing your baby's established bedtime routine and good sleep associations once they are healthy again.

Changes or disruptions, such as developmental milestones, traveling, or being taken care of by new people

New environments and unfamiliar people can be quite disruptive to your baby's sleep routine. If you notice that they are having trouble sleeping because of these factors, don't hesitate to comfort them more than usual.

Cut your baby some slack because they need time to adjust. Once they have gotten used to those changes or disruptions, ease them back into doing their usual bedtime routine again.

Trouble differentiating between day and night

Babies with this issue sleep a lot during the day but stay up beyond their supposed bedtime. This can be resolved without your intervention, but there are some ways to hasten this adjustment period.

For example, you can set a limit to how many naps your baby will get in a day. If your baby has been going for four 1-hour naps recently, try to shift them into having only three naps of the same length each day.

It also helps to further highlight the differences in their environment when it is daytime versus night-time. This can be as simple as drawing the curtains to keep their room as dark as possible or turning off the television whenever their bedtime routine is about to start.

Sleep regression isn't something that you can treat or drive away through sheer will. Instead of fixating on something immovable, focus on what you can do to reduce the impact or limit the effects of the prob-able triggers for sleep regression.

Remember to exercise patience and understanding during this period. This too shall pass!

Challenge #2: Overtiredness

We have already discussed overtiredness and its various signs across different age groups, but here's a quick recap of what it is and how it can affect your baby's sleep.

Overtiredness is the point between regular tiredness and total exhaustion. While babies can be ready to sleep when they feel tired, an overtired baby will resist doing so. Why?

It's beyond your baby's control. When they have reached the state of overtiredness, the natural balance within the body is disrupted and the stress response system kicks in. Stress hormones like cortisol and adrenaline will be released into their bloodstream.

In a normal situation, the presence of these hormones would prepare your body and mind for the "fight-or-flight" reaction. This means increased blood pressure, faster heart rate, and tensed muscles. Your mind becomes highly alert and aware of what's going on in your surroundings. All these things are necessary when you must face or run away from what is stressing you out.

Now, imagine your baby with their bloodstream flooded with stress hormones. Rather than give in to their fatigue, they will become even more agitated. If this happens again and again to your baby, it will lead to sleep deprivation.

You will know if your baby is suffering from sleep deprivation if:

- Their sleeping hours are below the average number of hours that a baby of their age should sleep in a day.
- They seem to resist the idea of going to sleep for no apparent reason.
- Even the slightest noises, such as the sound of a door opening, can easily startle them awake.
- During the daytime, their naps last for only 20 to 30 minutes.
- Sometimes they refuse to eat during the day, but somehow they eat a lot more than usual at night.
- They wake up frequently or stay asleep for far too long without waking up at night for their supposed feeding time.
- Making eye contact or smiling seems to be difficult for them.
- They exhibit a worried expression on their face.
- Their general mood is much better during the mornings compared to afternoons.
- As the day goes on, they find it harder and harder to fall asleep.
- They cry often, ranging from simple whining to inconsolable wails.

- Their attention span is very short.
- They want constant attention from their parents when they are awake.
- They tend to fuss even while you hold them in your arms, but will cry if you try to put them down.
- They dislike sitting or staying in their strollers, cribs, car seats, or highchairs.
- They prefer being rocked or swung around endlessly.
- They suffer extreme separation anxiety.
- They may fall asleep before they have finished eating.

Some of these signs are common behaviors exhibited by babies even when they are not sleep-deprived. Therefore, what you need to pay attention to is the degree and frequency to which your baby exhibits those behaviors. Be more observant of these signs when you know that your baby has not been getting enough sleep at night for their age.

If you ignore these signs, sleep deprivation can cause more problems for your baby. For example:

Overstimulation

This occurs when the nervous system receives too much sensory information at the same time. This can be particularly distressful for babies because they cannot remove themselves from the situation on their own. Newborns suffer the greatest because their nervous systems are not yet mature enough to process a lot of stimulation from their surroundings.

A sleep-deprived baby is more prone to suffering from overstimulation. As such, they will react strongly and negatively when they see bright lights; hear loud, sudden noises; or are touched or moved around. Upon reaching the point of overstimulation, a baby may cry for hours and hours, even when they are being soothed.

Gastrointestinal Discomfort

If you hear your baby fussing or crying out, one of the first causes that you might think of is that they are hungry. Naturally, this would prompt you to feed them to get them to stop crying.

However, whether you feed them with breastmilk or formula, there is a risk of causing them to suffer from gastrointestinal pain due to lactose overload. This refers to a problem that happens when babies are overfed. Their immature digestive system cannot handle too much milk, so it causes them to suffer from the following signs and symptoms:

- Bloating
- Stomach cramps
- Irritability
- Excessive farting
- "Explosive" bowel movements

Sleep-deprived babies cry a lot, so they are at great risk of gastrointestinal pain if their parents do not realize what is making them act out in the first place.

Fussy Feeding Behavior

When adults feel tired, their body coordination weakens, which can lead to frustrating situations. The same thing happens to babies whenever they feel physically fatigued.

In those cases, feeding becomes a struggle for babies. They will squirm, turn away from the nipple or the bottle, and refuse to eat, no matter if they are hungry or not. Some may give in and feed for a bit, but chances are, they will cough and splutter—or maybe even throw up what they have eaten so far. If you keep on pushing them, their fussing will soon devolve into screaming and crying.

Underfeeding

Sleep deprivation can make your baby feel too exhausted to continue feeding. Younger babies who need to wake up periodically at night to feed may no longer do so. Instead, they will sleep for an unusual amount of hours, even when they should be feeling hungry at that point.

If a baby continues to feed ineffectively for some time, the production of milk in the mother's breast will also drop. As a result, less and less breastmilk will be available for the baby in successive feedings. Though this may not be an issue for bottle-fed babies, those who have been fed breastmilk right from the start will find it even harder to feed themselves once the supply of breastmilk becomes insufficient for them.

Delays in Development

Exhaustion can prevent anyone from actively engaging in activities, retaining new information, and learning new skills. If a baby is frequently overtired to the point of chronic sleep deprivation, then they will likely have difficulties in developing their basic abilities.

This does not necessarily mean that these babies will not learn those things eventually. Instead, their rate of development is going to be much slower compared to those who regularly get enough high-quality sleep.

Misdiagnosis

Because of the probable negative effects that over-tiredness and sleep deprivation can cause for babies, some parents misdiagnose these conditions as something more serious, such as lactose intolerance, colic, or acid reflux.

As a result, those parents might push their babies to undergo dietary changes that they don't need and won't help in resolving the matter at all. Even worse, some might even consider giving their babies anti-colic or antacid medications, hoping that will effectively address the issue. Unfortunately, jumping to conclusions and misdiagnosing babies can only add to the distress that they are currently feeling, and in the long run, cause even bigger problems with their health.

Significant Distress on the Family

It's not just babies who will be negatively affected if they suffer from sleep deprivation every single day. Parents and other members of the family are likely to feel distressed upon seeing their precious little ones suffering from a lack of sleep. Moreover, taking care of babies falls under the responsibility of the older family members so they might see this as a failure to carry out their familial duties.

Babies tend to be either unresponsive or irritated when they feel overtired or sleep-deprived. This can strain the relationship between parent and child, especially when the parents don't understand why their babies are acting in that way.

Similarly, distressed parents can also take a colder or more aggressive approach when it comes to dealing with their babies' sleep issues. Even the gentlest people have their limits after all.

This could become a bigger problem if the parents are sleep-deprived, too. Your mood and judgment will be seriously impaired. Therefore, getting enough sleep is not just something that babies should have. Their parents must also have enough rest every day to keep their stress at a manageable level.

Keeping your baby from becoming overtired largely depends on how well you know their sleep associations and bedtime habits. Refer to the signs of tiredness and overtiredness across different age groups, as I shared earlier in this chapter. Observe which ones are exhibited by your baby and watch out for them whenever it is naptime or bedtime.

Encouraging Healthy Sleep Patterns for Your Baby

Sleep regression, overtiredness, and other sleep-related issues may plague you repeatedly as your baby continues to develop. Don't worry, plenty of other parents have gone through this before you, and survived these periods—some with great success.

After raising and sleep training my kids, I know how tough it can be to stay positive despite these challenges. That's why I'm sharing with you the things that I have done to accomplish my goal of guiding my children into adopting healthy sleep patterns, while also keeping me sane and happy.

Yes, it can get traumatic for parents like us—especially for first-timers—but you're never alone in trying to come up with good ways to resolve these issues.

Tip #1: Let your baby have their sleep associations.

This applies to 3- to 4-month-old babies who have not yet undergone sleep training. When they were in the newborn stage of development, chances are their sleep associations include bad ones such as being nursed or rocked to sleep.

If you have been doing that for the past few months to get your baby to sleep, continue to do it while your baby is experiencing sleep regression. After all, they have not learned any good sleep associations or better bedtime routines at this point.

You will have to wean them off of their sleep crutches once they start sleep training. For now, however, you can do whatever it takes to get your baby to sleep.

Tip #2: Stay consistent with your chosen sleep training method.

For those who have started sleep training their babies, the troubles caused by sleep regression or overtiredness are not an excuse for you to revert to relying on your baby's former sleep crutches. Yes, they can help immensely as a short-term option for putting your child to sleep. However, using them again would negate all the time and effort you have put forth so far in sleep training your baby.

Try your best to remain consistent with your plan and established bedtime routine. Since you have started laying your baby down when they are just drowsy, continue to do so even when they fuss or cry more than usual.

You may need to provide extra comfort to get your baby to sleep, especially during periods of sleep regression. That's perfectly okay. However, avoid doing things that are considered bad sleep associations, such as picking up your baby whenever they cry or rocking them in your arms until they fall asleep again.

Remember: Consistency is key. Your shortcuts will work now, but in the long run, they won't do you or your baby any good. Think of these challenging nights as more opportunities for your baby to learn how to self-soothe and sleep on their own.

Tip #3: Consider adjusting your baby's sleep schedule.

Sleep regressions can lead to overtiredness since some babies skip their naptimes during the day. This can go on for several days, thus causing you and your child to suffer from sleep deprivation.

If your baby has fewer daytime naps, you might have to adjust their bedtime to an earlier hour. This will keep them from being so exhausted that they become overtired. Remember to stick to your baby's bedtime routine though, even if you change their sleep schedule.

Tip #4: Improve your baby's nap schedule.

Taking naps during the day helps babies a lot, especially when it comes to encouraging them to adopt healthy sleep patterns. By having enough sleep in the daytime, your baby will have a lower risk of becoming overtired. They will more likely go to bed at the right time each night, and stay asleep for the rest of the night.

Studies also show that naps can be a great mood booster (Fry, 2020). They help in regulating emotions as well as recharging one's energy level.

A good nap schedule is consistent and never goes beyond 4 p.m. You will learn more about the optimal sleep schedule for babies in the next chapter. In general, however, two to three naps that last for the same amount of time would be enough for most babies.

When my child Alex was 10 months old, his first naptime was at 10 in the morning, while the next one was at 2 in the afternoon. Each nap lasted for 1 hour. Through this, we were able to follow his usual bedtime schedule, even when he started taking his first steps around the same time.

Tip #5: Consider that there might be delays or interruptions in your baby's sleep schedule.

Certain things in life cannot be entirely avoided, no matter how much you plan every day. Sometimes, appointments cannot be canceled—or they may have gone longer than expected—thus preventing you from letting your baby nap on time.

There are also days when you just cannot seem to get your baby to settle well enough for them to go to sleep. It may be because your baby is feeling too much excitement during the day, or they might be feeling unwell due to an illness or pain.

Whatever the reason may be, you must learn how to read the sleep cues of your baby instead of just fixating on a specific time. You may be putting your child to bed by 8 p.m. every day, but that does not mean that it must be that way all the time. Be observant of their facial expressions and gestures to see if you need to make their bedtime earlier on certain days. This will keep them from feeling overtired and losing their precious sleep.

Tip #6: Don't feel bad for feeling frustrated.

Sleep training your baby takes time, and so does encouraging them to follow healthier sleep patterns. You can't expect long-lasting results when you have worked on it for just a few nights.

Listening to your baby fuss, scream, and cry can be incredibly frustrating since you are not allowed to intervene unless the situation is endangering your baby's safety. However, if you are certain that your little one has been well-fed and changed before bed, and that they are not sick or injured, then you can put your mind at ease that the distress they are feeling right now is just temporary. Believe that your baby can make themselves stop crying and go to sleep on their own.

Tip #7: Turn to your partner, a family member, or a friend for help.

As I have said in previous chapters, sleep training your baby is not a project that you must bear all on your own. Hearing your baby fuss and cry night after night can take a toll on your well-being, too.

You can minimize these negative effects by asking others to join you in sleep training your baby. Discuss with them how to divide the responsibilities involved, as well as your expectations from one another.

Some parents opt to handle things on alternate days. Others assign one to daytime naps while their partners take over for nighttime sleep.

Do whatever would work for everyone involved. It also helps if sleep training is regarded not as a task or chore, but as an opportunity to bond with your baby and make them feel loved and secure.

In terms of managing the other aspects of your household, seek the help of your friends or other family members who can take over some of the things that you don't have the energy left to do. Perhaps your parents or siblings can drop by and help you prepare and cook meals. Or maybe your friends could help by doing some general cleaning around the house.

Reach out to those who care for you and your baby. Those who have kids of their own are likely to know what you are going through.

Fostering healthy sleep patterns for your baby requires understanding, patience, and consistency. There are not inherently good or bad sleepers among babies. You, as their parent, can mold their habits and preferences into something that will enable them and everyone else in the family to have restful nights.

We have touched on several things that you can do to accomplish this goal—one of which is napping. Your sleep training approach is not holistic if you will not work on improving the way your baby naps as well. It's connected to how well they sleep at night, so in the following chapter, we shall focus on how you can harness the benefits of naps to fully shift your baby's sleep pattern into a healthy and sustainable one.

6

DAYS 6 AND 7: THE HOME STRETCH

For the last two days of sleep training your baby, the key component is consistency. What you have set out to do during the first few days should still be in place up to Day 7. This means your baby's bedtime routine must be carried out just as it has for the previous days, and you must leave your baby in their crib while they are drowsy but not yet asleep.

Just like in Day 4 and Day 5, the changes in the last two days of sleep training are in the pre-determined waiting times until your baby has completely fallen to sleep. As a guide, look below for my suggested waiting times for Day 6 and Day 7 of the gradual extinction training plan:

Day 6

- Initial Waiting Time: 17 minutes
- Second Waiting Time: 20 minutes
- Succeeding Waiting Time: 25 minutes

Day 7

- Initial Waiting Time: 20 minutes
- Second Waiting Time: 25 minutes
- Succeeding Waiting Time: 30 minutes

The increasing time intervals for each day will give your baby more of an opportunity to practice what they have learned so far. It's also enough time for them to figure out which of their self-chosen methods to soothe themselves will be most effective for them. By the end of Day 7, you should be reassured that your baby can fall asleep, stay asleep, and go back to sleep with no help from you anymore.

To ensure the success of the last two days of sleep training, you should turn your focus to optimizing the nap schedule, as well as addressing their feelings of anxiety whenever you leave them alone. We will also tackle what else you should do once you have completely sleep-trained your baby.

Setting Up the Ideal Naptime for Your Baby

How many naps should your baby have in a day? And how long should each nap be?

The answer differs according to your baby's age and current development. Though no one answer is guaranteed to work for every baby, aim to at least let your baby have a 1-hour nap each day—provided they are not younger than 4 months old.

When your baby reaches 6 months of age, they should have at least two 1-hour naps or longer. As they grow older, babies will transition to one nap only, but make sure that it lasts for around 2 to 3 hours.

To better guide you on the optimal nap schedule for your baby, I'm sharing these nap guidelines for babies across different age groups.

0 to 11 Weeks

- Number of Naps: 6 to 8
- Duration of Each Nap: 10 to 15 minutes
- Interval Between Each Nap: 30 minutes to 1 hour
- Total Daytime Nap Hours: 4 to 5 hours

At this age, naps can be short and irregular, so don't panic if your baby seems to be sleeping shorter or longer than expected. Rather than focusing solely on your newborn's nap schedule, consider their feeding schedule and sleep routines to plan out how the other activities of your baby should go.

3 to 4 Months

- Number of Naps: 4 to 5
- Duration of Each Nap: 3o minutes to 2 hours
- Interval Between Each Nap: 1 to 2 hours
- Total Daytime Nap Hours: 3 to 4 hours

Napping can become a complicated affair for babies in this age group if they experience sleep regression.

5 to 6 Months

- Number of Naps: 3 to 4
- Duration of Each Nap: 30 or 45 minutes to 2 hours
- Interval Between Each Nap: around 2 hours
- Total Daytime Nap Hours: 2.5 to 3.5 hours

During the previous ages, shorter naps are the norm for babies. However, upon reaching this age, your baby's nap will gradually become longer and more predictable.

7 to 8 Months

- Number of Naps: 2 to 3
- Duration of Each Nap: 1 to 2 hours
- Interval Between Each Nap: 2 to 3 hours
- Total Daytime Nap Hours: 2 to 3 hours

Expect another round of sleep regression to occur in your baby's eighth month. Many babies also begin their nap transition at this age, going from three naps a day down to only two.

9 to 12 Months

- Number of Naps: 2
- Duration of Each Nap: 1 to 2 hours
- Interval Between Each Nap: 3 to 4 hours
- Total Daytime Nap Hours: 2 to 3 hours

In general, the nap schedules of babies who belong to this age group are quite predictable. If your baby isn't, evaluate their feeding schedule and see if there are any adjustments to be made. Feeding should be less frequent by now since your baby has been eating solid foods instead of just breastmilk or formula.

13 to 14 Months

- Number of Naps: 1 to 2
- Duration of Each Nap: 1 to 3 hours
- Interval Between Each Nap: 3 to 5 hours
- Total Daytime Nap Hours: 2 to 3 hours

Refrain from pushing your baby into another nap transition, where they would only need to nap once a day. Let it happen naturally—some babies transition early, but many will do so by their fifteenth to eighteenth month of age.

15 to 18 Months

- Number of Naps: 1 to 2
- Duration of Each Nap: 1 to 3 hours
- Interval Between Each Nap: 4 to 5 hours
- Total Daytime Nap Hours: 2 to 3 hours

This is the ideal time to encourage your baby to transition to only one nap each day. You can do this by adjusting their feeding schedule again.

18 to 24 Months

- Number of Naps: 1
- Duration of Each Nap: 2 to 3 hours
- Interval Between Each Nap: 5 to 5.5 hours
- Total Daytime Nap Hours: 2 to 3 hours

Be mindful of the interval between the end of your toddler's afternoon nap and their supposed bedtime. As they grow older, toddlers need to have a longer wake time in the afternoon. If you let them nap too late in the day, you will also have to push back their bedtime to a later hour.

You don't have to exactly follow the frequency and duration in the baby nap guidelines above. After all, your baby's needs and rate of development are unique.

Try them out first, and then observe if the schedule agrees with your baby. If not, feel free to adjust until you have figured out the optimal nap schedule for your little one.

Dealing with Your Baby's Separation Anxiety

As I said in the previous chapter, separation anxiety among babies is quite common. It's a natural part of their development, and if handled well, it may lead to a stronger and healthier bond between parents and their babies.

This does not mean that you just must bear seeing your child transform into a screaming, crying, and clingy mess every time you leave them alone, even for just two minutes. There are plenty of ways to effectively reassure them during this period and ease them into embracing the new abilities that allow them to be somewhat independent of you.

To better manage your baby's separation anxiety, you need to understand why it happens in the first place. According to sleep experts, two important milestones occur during a baby's seventh or eighth month and are primarily responsible for this.

A. Better ability to distinguish one person from another

During the first few months after birth, most babies cannot tell one person apart from another. To them, everyone seems to look and feel the same. As such, these babies do not mind being held or taken care of by different people.

Things may drastically change once babies reach the point of their development where they can recognize the person who is with them. Typically, their attachments will become stronger toward their parents, or whoever is primarily taking care of them.

While this can be a sign of healthy social development, it can pose a problem when your baby cannot stand the thought of being left in the care of other people. Even if they used to enjoy the company of others, your baby may no longer feel that way once they realize that you and those people are not the same.

B. Learning the concept of object permanence

Babies who understand object permanence know that a person or an object doesn't stop existing just because they do not see them anymore.

It's not something you can teach or train them to do though. Around the seventh or eighth month, most babies will develop this ability. That's why simple games like peek-a-boo are much more entertaining for younger babies. They believe anything that is not in their line of sight has somehow disappeared and its reappearance seems magical to them.

How does object permanence lead to separation anxiety though?

When your baby is younger, leaving their room puts you out of their sight and out of their mind. You simply do not exist for them anymore.

However, once babies have learned object permanence, they will realize that you are just somewhere else. However, they do not have a good sense of time yet. And if they have not yet learned that you may return to them at some point, such thoughts will lead to separation anxiety.

If your baby is around 6 to 10 months old, pay attention to how they react whenever you leave them in the company of other people, or during bedtime or naptime.

Separation anxiety does not happen gradually. Often, it takes parents by surprise, which then makes them feel panicked that something is wrong with their babies.

Aside from being a pain when it comes to social situations, separation anxiety can also negatively affect your baby's sleep. Feeling anxious about their parent's lack of presence will make it harder for them to settle and self-soothe. As a result, their resistance to sleep or nap may lead to overtiredness and eventually, sleep deprivation.

If your baby is experiencing separation anxiety, the first thing you should do is acknowledge the validity of her feelings, doubts, and fears. Their cries and clinginess aren't tricks to get what they want. Believing otherwise can not only cause them more sleep-related problems, but also attachment issues.

Take Note!

Separation anxiety may be one of the factors that can cause your baby to suffer from sleep regression. It may also become better or worse as your baby grows older.

While you cannot do anything to make sleep regression "go away" faster, you may deal with your baby's separation anxiety by focusing instead on making your baby feel loved and secured even when you must leave them on their own, or with other people.

Minimizing the likelihood of having separation anxiety—or at least lessening its intensity—is something that you can do for your baby if they are not yet in the middle of it. Here are some ideas that you can try practicing with your baby:

Play games that involve you hiding and then reappearing before them.

Popular examples of such games include peek-a-boo —for younger babies—and hide-and-seek for older ones. Most babies enjoy these games a lot, even if you frequently and repeatedly do it with them.

Make it a point to hide your face or yourself for a little bit longer each time. If you have enough space, vary your hiding spots, too. Observe how far you can take things as you gradually push your baby's limits when it comes to not seeing you.

Toddlers find the idea of hiding themselves entertaining as well. They like the challenge and the excitement that this activity brings them.

By playing games like these often, you are slowly letting your child get used to the idea that they will see you again after you have left them for whatever reason.

Show your baby what you will be doing while they are asleep.

Though babies can't communicate well enough to discuss things with you, a study shows that they understand the things shown to them more than expected (Pathman & Bauer, 2020).

For example, as part of my second baby's bedtime routine, we would briefly go to my bedroom to show her that I would be staying there while she slept. If I was staying up late for work reasons, we would head to our study or the living room instead. I'd talk to her for a bit about my plans for the night and then proceed with the other activities in her bedtime routine.

While I didn't know for sure if she understood what I was doing at the time, it helped in settling her down for bed and reassuring her that I was nearby whenever she woke up in the middle of the night.

Let your baby get used to the idea of being taken care of by people other than you.

I have advised this often across different chapters of this book. As much as possible, involve other people in the sleep routine of your baby. Doing this can help them understand that they don't need to be with you all the time just to feel safe and comfortable.

Of course, if you are breastfeeding your baby, then you will likely be the only person who would be putting them to bed every night. However, once you have stopped nursing them to sleep, ask someone else to take part in your baby's bedtime routine.

If your baby is already experiencing separation anxiety, then you should deal with it by rebuilding their confidence that they are loved and cared for even if you are not physically present beside them. Below are some helpful tips that worked well with my children before:

Tip #1: Take a positive approach.

As heartbreaking it is to see your baby clinging to you with tears in their eyes, refrain from going along with their emotions. Avoid crying yourself or showing them an anxious facial expression. Otherwise, you are essentially telling them that there is something to be worried about when the two of you are not together.

Stay positive and keep things light, especially during naptime or bedtime. Your relaxed disposition and calm demeanor will help make your baby feel the same way, too.

"The best baby-sitters, of course, are the baby's grandparents. You feel completely comfortable entrusting your baby to them for long periods, which is why most grandparents flee to Florida."

— DAVE BARRY

Tip #2: Sneaking away isn't the answer.

We joke about moving like a ninja when babies are trying to sleep. While moving around quietly can help them settle quicker, sneaking away from your baby could do more harm than good.

If you make it a habit to leave your baby's room when they are distracted, you are unconsciously feeding their worries about not seeing you. It reinforces the idea that they should not look away from you at all. Otherwise, you are going to vanish and leave them on their own.

Instead of sneaking away, let your baby know and see that you are about to head out of their room. Bid them a goodnight coupled with a few loving and gentle touches. Say some reassuring words even if they cannot understand what you mean yet—sometimes even just the tone of your voice can help ease their anxieties.

"That moment when you go to check on your sleeping baby and their eyes ping open so you drop to the floor and roll out of the room like a ninja."

— UNKNOWN

Tip #3: Provide comfort to your baby when they need it, but don't overdo it.

If your baby's separation anxiety is making them scream and cry hard, do not hesitate to offer them comfort. Just make sure that your chosen method isn't going to create new sleep crutches.

As before, your main goal for comforting your baby is to reassure them that you are close by. You don't have to stay until they have fallen asleep though. It is best to keep this short but sweet—nothing too lively that it excites rather than relaxes them.

This means no singing of lullabies, bedtime games, or reading books together. Say a few words, give them gentle but brief pats, and then leave their room again. Staying for too long might undo the progress you have made so far in guiding them into sleeping on their own.

Tip #4: Keep your promises.

This one is more applicable to older babies who understand the concept of promises. When my daughter Kate was around 24 months old, her separation anxiety came back with a vengeance. It threw off her sleep schedule, even though I had already sleep-trained her before.

To build back her confidence, I made it a point to promise her that I would be back soon to check on her before leaving her bedroom on the first night of my intervention. After about two minutes, I returned as promised—thereby showing her that my reassurances were not just words.

Doing this a couple more times was enough to calm her fears, and after some time, Kate was able to go to sleep even before I had headed back to her room to fulfill my promise.

Guiding your baby through their separation anxiety requires patience and understanding. Don't invalidate their feelings, especially since they can't vocalize them yet. Instead, let them feel secure and confident that you will always be there for them when they need you.

Congratulations on Completing the Seven-Day Sleep Training Plan! Now, What?

So, let's say that you have already successfully sleep-trained your little one. They can fall to sleep on their own during bedtime. Staying asleep is no longer an issue—waking up only when it's time for their next feed, or when it is the next morning already.

You're thinking that with your baby peacefully dreaming away, you can now catch up on your sleep. After all, you deserve this much at least, right?

Not every parent gets to reap such a reward.

Sometimes, babies tend to wake up as soon as the sun rises in the morning—or even before then. No matter how quiet and relaxing their surroundings are, they will wake up when the rest of the family isn't quite ready to leave the bed yet.

Don't despair though! I have some tips for that too.

"Why don't kids understand that their nap is not for them but for us?"

— ALYSON HANNIGAN

There's a chance that all of the following won't work well for you, but each one is worth trying, just so you can enjoy a few more minutes—or maybe even hours—in bed.

Tip #1: Make sure that your baby's bedroom stays quiet and dim, even in the morning.

Mimic how their surroundings are when they go to sleep. That means reducing the amount of light that can enter their room, while also dampening any sound that may be coming in from the outside.

Those who are trying to save money can do this by placing a thick blanket over the window of their baby's bedroom. However, if you have some budget to spare, consider investing in heavy, sound-muffling shades instead.

Tip #2: Adjust their nap and sleep schedule.

Try to move the naptimes and bedtime of your baby to find the sweet spot for everyone in the family. While bedtimes set to a later time seem to be the obvious choice when it comes to encouraging your baby to sleep in, earlier bedtimes may be the answer for some.

For example, if your baby tends to wake up at dawn and refuses to go back to sleep, then they might be feeling overtired by the time they go to sleep. Giving your baby a chance to have more rest by setting an earlier bedtime may be the key to breaking them out of this unhealthy pattern.

Remember to consider adjusting your baby's naps, too. Extra daytime napping can push back their bedtime to a later hour, while limiting their nap frequency or duration may require you to put your baby to sleep at an earlier time.

Tip #3: Provide entertainment or comfort through baby-safe toys.

This strategy applies more to babies who are at least 7 months old. By then, there is far less risk of your baby choking or being smothered by toys placed inside their crib.

Popular choices of baby-safe toys include stuffed animal toys and cloth books. If you are not comfortable with this idea, placing a mirror where your baby can see their reflection may be entertaining enough for them without the added risk brought about by having certain toys within reach.

Feel free to experiment to figure out which ones grab the attention and pique the interest of your baby. If you manage to do so, then you can sleep in in the morning while they entertain themselves on their own.

Tip #4: Wait.

Many parents seem to be hard-wired to react immediately whenever they see or hear signs that their babies have woken up. If you want to have extra time in bed during the mornings, refrain from acting upon those impulses immediately.

Take your time and observe them for a few minutes. Sometimes, babies will fall back to sleep on their own if they do not receive any attention when they wake up.

With these tips, you might be able to enjoy your hard-earned sleep without worrying too much about the following morning. Yes, these are not fool-proof ideas, but as long as you are not causing irreparable and irrevocable harm to your baby, consider practicing the ideas I have shared with you in this chapter.

CONCLUSION

There's a popular quote that goes, "A baby makes love stronger, the days shorter, the nights longer, savings smaller, and a home happier."

I quite agree with the sentiment behind these words. However, as you have learned in this book, you don't have to settle for shorter days and longer nights. Sleep training can be an effective way to resolve the problems and pains brought about by your baby's sleep issues.

It's not a one-size-fits-all solution, but don't you think it's worth giving a try?

At its core, sleep training requires parents to be consistent, persistent, and patient as their babies adjust to healthier and more sustainable sleep patterns. There are no bells and whistles involved but you must be careful and thoughtful while planning it out.

Once you have established the right bedtime routine for your baby, all you have to do is wait outside their bedroom, look out for signs of extreme discomfort, and provide some comfort when needed until your baby falls asleep.

Yes, it sounds easier said than done. But with the tips and techniques I have shared with you in this book, I hope to help you start on the right foot, and prepare you to face and overcome the challenges along the way.

I'd like to highlight this key takeaway point that might have been lost amidst the volume of new information you have learned from reading this book: Be mindful of your current mood and attitude toward sleep and sleep training.

As I explained earlier, babies are like mirrors of the people around them. If your baby sees you frowning or crying along with them during bedtime, chances are they will feel even more upset. Learn to control your emotions and take a step back from sleep training your baby, if needed.

This is why I insist on involving friends or other members of the family in taking care of your child. Their support and encouragement can be the boost you need to keep going toward your goal to improve the way your baby sleeps.

Your next step is to put the things you have learned into action. I hope that you have carefully read each chapter so that you can be guided all the way from planning your baby's sleep training up to completing the seven-day program. If you have anything to clarify or share about the many points covered here, feel free to send them my way in your review of this book on whatever platform you purchased it from. I read all of my readers' reviews and I use them to make relevant content for your lives. Let me know how I did! Share a success story or your unique struggles. I hope to hear from all of you.

Once again, I hope that by reading through my several years' worth of experience about sleep training, you now feel more confident to go after your ultimate goal of ensuring that everyone in your family will sleep well throughout the night.

I hope you've had a great time reading this book! And if you found the content valuable or helpful, I'd greatly appreciate it if you would leave a review on Amazon or Audible telling others about your experience. I read every review, and they are extremely valuable to a caring author like me. Thank you, and I wish you a good night's sleep!

REFERENCES

Benoit, D. (2004, October 1). *Infant-parent attachment: Definition, types, antecedents, measurement and outcome.* PubMed Central (PMC). https://www.ncbi.nlm.nih.gov/pmc/articles/PMC2724160/

Burnham, M., Goodlin-Jones, B., Gaylor, E., & Anders, T. (2002, September 1). *Nighttime sleep-wake patterns and self-soothing from birth to one year of age: A longitudinal intervention study.* PubMed Central (PMC). https://www.ncbi.nlm.nih.gov/pmc/articles/PMC1201415/

Canapari, C. (2021, May 5). *The top ten sleep training mistakes (and how To avoid them).* Craig Canapari, MD. https://drcraigcanapari.com/sleep-training-mistakes-and-pitfalls/

Dahl, R. (2007, September 1). *Sleep and the developing brain*. PubMed Central (PMC). https://www.ncbi. nlm.nih.gov/pmc/articles/PMC1978403/

Fry, A. (2020, October 9). *Napping*. Sleep Foundation. https://www.sleepfoundation.org/sleep-hygiene/napping

Gradisar, M. (2016, May 21). *Behavioral interventions for infant sleep problems: A randomized controlled trial*. American Academy of Pediatrics. https://pediatrics. aappublications.org/content/early/2016/05/21/ peds.2015-1486?sso=1&sso_redirect_count=3& nfstatus=401&nftoken=00000000-0000-0000- 0000-000000000000&nfstatusdescription= ERROR%3A%20No%20local%20token&nfstatus= 401&nftoken=00000000-0000-0000-0000- 000000000000&nfstatusdescription=ERROR%3a+ No+local+token

Hiscock, H., Bayer, J., Gold, L., Hampton, A., Ukoumunne, O., & Wake, M. (2007, November 1). *Improving infant sleep and maternal mental health: A cluster randomised trial*. PubMed Central (PMC). https://www.ncbi.nlm.nih.gov/pmc/ articles/PMC2083609/

Lewis, P. M., & Granic, P. I. (2010). *Bedtiming: The parent's guide to getting your child to sleep at just the right age*. The Experiment. My Book

Nahidi, F., Gazerani, N., Yousefi, P., & Abadi, A. R. (2017). *The comparison of the effects of massaging and rocking on infantile colic*. PubMed Central (PMC). https://www.ncbi.nlm.nih.gov/pmc/articles/PMC5364756/

Pacheco, D. (2021, January 15). *Bedtime routines for children*. Sleep Foundation. https://www.sleepfoundation.org/children-and-sleep/bedtime-routine#:%7E:text=A%20predictable%20routine%20also%20gives,up%20less%20during%20the%20night.

Pathman, T., & Bauer, P. (2020). *Brain | Memory and early brain development*. Encyclopedia on Early Childhood Development. https://www.child-encyclopedia.com/brain/according-experts/memory-and-early-brain-development

Reilly J. J., Armstrong J., Dorosty, A.R., et al. *Early life risk factors for obesity in childhood: Cohort study.* PubMed. https://pubmed.ncbi.nlm.nih.gov/15908441/

Sadler, S. (1994). *Sleep: What is normal at six months?* PubMed. https://pubmed.ncbi.nlm. nih.gov/8680184/

Simard, V. (2008). *Longitudinal study of preschool sleep disturbance: The predictive role of maladaptive parental behaviors, early sleep problems, and child/mother psychological factors.* PubMed. https://pubmed.ncbi.nlm. nih.gov/18391145/

Weissbluth, M. (2015). *Healthy sleep habits, happy child: A step-by-step program for a good night's sleep* (4th ed.). Ballantine Books. My Book